BACK PAIN RELIEF PLAN

A 20-MINUTE EXERCISE-BASED PROGRAM TO PREVENT, MANAGE, AND EASE PAIN

RICKY FISHMAN, DC

Illustrations by Christy Ni

ROCKRIDGE
PRESS

For general information on our other products and services or to obtain technical support, please contact our Customer Care Department within the United States at (866) 744-2665, or outside the United States at (510) 253-0500.

Rockridge Press publishes its books in a variety of electronic and print formats. Some content that appears in print may not be available in electronic books, and vice versa.

TRADEMARKS: Rockridge Press and the Rockridge Press logo are trademarks or registered trademarks of Callisto Media Inc. and/or its affiliates, in the United States and other countries, and may not be used without written permission. All other trademarks are the property of their respective owners. Rockridge Press is not associated with any product or vendor mentioned in this book.

Interior and Cover Designer: Lindsey Dekker
Art Producer: Janice Ackerman
Editor: Sean Newcott
Production Manager: Michael Kay
Production Editor: Melissa Edeburn
Illustrations © Christy Ni, 2021

ISBN: Print 978-1-64739-233-8 | eBook 978-1-64739-234-5
R0

To every patient I have treated through my many years of practice. Thank you for sharing your healing journeys with me.

Contents

Introduction ix

PART I: UNDERSTANDING YOUR BACK 1

CHAPTER 1: The Backstory on Pain 5

CHAPTER 2: Diagnosis and Treatment 17

CHAPTER 3: Habits for a Healthy Back 29

PART II: THE BACK PAIN ACTION PLAN 41

CHAPTER 4: Workout Programs 43

CHAPTER 5: Stretching 51

CHAPTER 6: Strengthening 71

Epilogue 141

Resources 142

References 144

Index 146

Introduction

From an early age, I had a powerful calling to become a healer. I could always instinctively sense what other people were feeling—their happiness and joy, but also their suffering. When I discovered the world of chiropractic medicine, I found a system of healing that allowed me to actually do something about people's pain. I could make their lives better using only my hands and my mind.

Chiropractic care is very effective for treating back pain. Almost all the patients I saw in my office were suffering from back pain, so treating it became a central focus of my work. And I'm glad it did.

Early in my career, I offered my clients standard chiropractic adjustments. I performed spinal manipulations that helped relieve their nerve irritation and stop their pain, but often only temporarily. Some patients had to see me repeatedly, which was not what I wanted. I needed to understand why their pain persisted and figure out how to give them the tools to stop the pain from returning.

Through my decades of practice and research I've found one simple truth: For many people, regardless of what's causing their back pain, the most effective remedy is to build a strong and flexible body through stretching and exercise.

My goal with *The Back Pain Relief Plan* is to provide you (or a friend, a loved one, or anyone else you know who is living with back pain) with a customizable pain-relieving training program. I am pleased to be able to share with you the safe, effective training program I've worked to develop with my patients. My program focuses on the lower back, the most common area of pain and discomfort, but you can use it to treat the rest of your back as well.

This book lays out a series of exercises, stretches, and low-impact cardio workouts that range from easy to hard. In addition, it makes recommendations about diet, sleep, and workspace ergonomics.

When you're in pain, it can be hard to imagine life without it, especially if your pain comes and goes—just when you think you've moved past it, it's back. I know all about that frustration, but there is hope. When you are experiencing your worst pain, know that countless people have defeated their own back pain with a smart, consistent stretching and exercise program.

I encourage you to absorb the information in this book. Once you understand why you have back pain, you can get to work on treating it.

You possess incredible healing power, but it takes courage and fortitude to tap into it. I hope this book helps you find that power and sets you off on your journey toward a life without back pain.

PART I

UNDERSTANDING YOUR BACK

Lower back pain is one of the most common health problems that brings people into their doctor's office. This pain doesn't discriminate. It affects both young and old, people who are otherwise totally healthy and those with preexisting conditions, workers who sit at computers all day and those who drive forklifts or work in factories.

These statistics from the American Chiropractic Association illuminate the scope of the back pain problem:

- Approximately 31 million Americans—nearly 1 in 10—are experiencing lower back pain at any given time.

- Back pain is the leading cause of disability, preventing many people from engaging in work and everyday activities.

- From 1990 to 2015, disability claims relating to back pain increased by 54 percent.

- Approximately 80 percent of the population will experience back pain during their lifetimes.

- Each year, lower back pain costs Americans at least $50 billion, not including lost wages and decreased productivity.

To understand why back pain, and particularly lower back pain, is so widespread today, travel back in history with me. Roughly 25,000 years ago, humans had the same basic bodies we have today. It took hundreds of thousands of years for the human form to evolve to support tremendously active lives: walking every day in search of food, chasing animals (and occasionally running from them), climbing trees to gather fruit, and digging into the ground to find edible roots.

The human body is no longer in sync with modern times. Many individuals have lost strength as a result of a sedentary lifestyle. Others have occupations that require them to perform repetitive physical tasks that put a great deal of strain on the lower back. In both cases, the human body is working in a way it was not evolved to.

Lower back pain in particular is on the rise. Like so many chronic conditions, including diabetes and heart disease, lower back pain is usually the product of a perfect storm of modern factors: eating poorly, packing on extra pounds, not getting enough sleep, spending too much time sitting around, not having the time and energy to exercise, and feeling overloaded by stress.

There are many types of lower back pain. Individuals experience differences in intensity, from dull and achy to burning and sharp. Some people experience pain after an accident, whereas pain develops gradually for others.

No matter the cause, all back pain falls into one of three categories: acute, subacute, or chronic.

Acute. This type of back pain is the most common. Almost everyone experiences it at some point, even if they are in good overall physical health. Acute pain comes on suddenly and strongly and generally goes away with basic self-care.

Subacute. Pain that lasts longer than six weeks is categorized as subacute. The quality of the pain may change from sharp and burning to achy and dull, but it is persistent.

Chronic. Beyond 12 weeks, back pain is considered chronic.

The right treatment generally depends on which type of pain you have. Before diving into the specific action plans to treat your pain, it's helpful to have a good understanding of your back, including the muscles and tendons, ligaments and discs, nerves and blood vessels. Before you can treat your back, you have to find the root of your pain.

CHAPTER 1

The Backstory on Pain

Even though back pain is very common, it's not always easy to pinpoint its causes. The lower back is very complex. A lot of body parts work together to create a finely tuned machine. As with most machines, however, if any piece is broken, worn, or out of alignment, it will impact the other components, setting off a chain reaction of malfunctions that will prevent the lower back from performing correctly.

Back treatment is tricky because most people don't have any idea they have a problem until they feel pain, and in many cases the discomfort is far downstream from its original source. For example, you might spend too many hours sitting at your desk, which causes your lower back muscles and joints to tighten up, which then irritates your nerves, which are actually causing the pain.

One final note before we dive into the anatomy lesson: I lay out as much as I can here to help you zero in on the source of your back pain so you can follow the safest and most effective exercise plan. As you listen to your body, however, you may find that you want or need a professional to do the detective work and help you figure out the right course of action for your unique needs.

Anatomy Lesson

Each structure that makes up the back is essential for proper function, but each can also be a potential source of pain and dysfunction.

Vertebrae. The vertebrae, or bones of the spine, work together to make up the spinal column. There are several groups of vertebrae, with 24 in total: 7 make up the neck (cervical spine), 12 make up the middle back (thoracic spine), and 5 make up the lower back (lumbar spine).

The sacrum, which connects to your lowest lumbar region, is made of five vertebrae that fused together early in life. And, finally, connected to the sacrum is the tailbone (also known as the coccyx).

Pelvis. The pelvis is made up of three fused bones: ischium, ilium, and pubis. The sacrum connects to the ilium at the sacroiliac joint. This joint is often involved in lower back pain and dysfunction.

Discs. Spinal discs (or intervertebral discs) are the soft-tissue cushions between the vertebrae. Each disc is made up of two main parts: The tough, fibrous outer part is the annulus fibrosus, and the watery, gelatinous inner part is the nucleus pulposus. The discs act like shock absorbers, helping distribute normal and traumatic forces that come through the spine. The discs work with your vertebrae to allow for large bending movements. They also make up one part of the intervertebral foramen, the space through which the spinal nerves travel. This space is bounded by both the discs and the vertebrae.

Muscles and tendons. Your back muscles and tendons act as stabilizers for your spinal joints and are responsible for how you can move your back. Your tendons are the soft tissue that connect your muscles to your bones.

Muscles are rich in blood supply because they use quite a bit of energy to contract and create movement, which produces natural waste products. These normal products of muscular metabolism include biological acids. If these acids aren't efficiently swept away, they can contribute to back pain.

Tendons are made of tough, fibrous connective tissue designed to stabilize structures, not move them. Because tendons don't contract like muscles, they don't require a heavy blood supply. The difference in blood supply between muscles and tendons is significant when it comes to the healing of injuries.

Ligaments. Like tendons, ligaments are a kind of connective tissue. They're very tough and attach bone to bone to stabilize joints. Wherever one vertebra forms a joint with the one above or below it, it is secured and stabilized by ligaments.

Nerves. The nerves throughout your back (and the rest of your body) are extensions of your central nervous system. This system starts in your brain and continues through your spinal cord, which is protected by the bony spinal column. The spinal cord then branches off into nerve roots that exit the spine as spinal nerves. These nerves form a web that connects to every structure in your body.

This book focuses on two different types of nerves: motor and sensory. Motor nerves send out signals to act. For example, if you want to bend your elbow, this simple act requires a lot of action behind the scenes. First, you formulate the thought in your brain, then the brain sends a message through the spinal cord to the spinal nerve. This message reaches the biceps muscle, which is responsible for bending. The biceps contracts, and your elbow bends.

Sensory nerve endings, on the other hand, are embedded in vertebrae, muscles, ligaments, tendons, discs, and the rest of the body. These nerves react to different kinds of stimulation and send signals back along the spinal nerve to the spinal cord and up to the brain. The brain receives the signal and interprets it based on the type of stimulation. For example, receiving a back massage could produce positive sensations like feelings of well-being and relaxation. Falling off a ladder and landing with blunt force will stimulate the nerve endings to produce feelings of sharp and throbbing pain.

Intervertebral joint complex. While it is important to know the anatomy of the structures described above, it also helps to understand how all the parts work together. They are not just individual pieces, but parts that make up a complex, highly functional system.

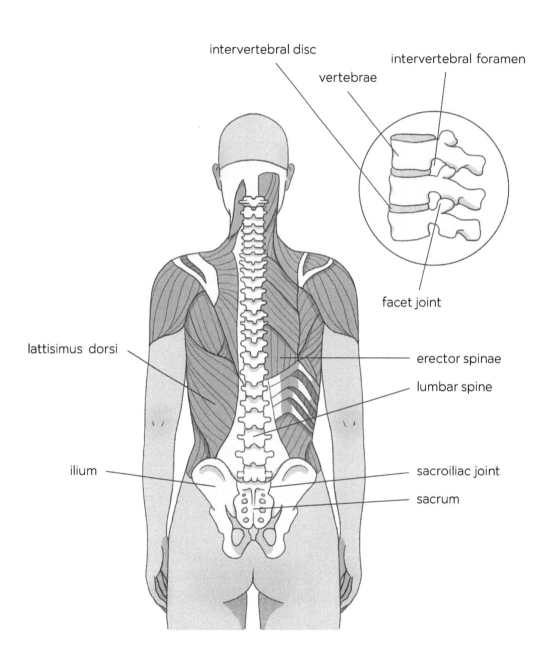

intervertebral disc

vertebrae

intervertebral foramen

facet joint

lattisimus dorsi

erector spinae

lumbar spine

ilium

sacroiliac joint

sacrum

Vertebrae are connected to each other in different ways. In the front (anterior), vertebrae are connected by the disc that separates them; in the back (posterior), they're connected by facets. Together, they make up the intervertebral joint. Injury to the anterior or posterior part of the joint usually has different causes and will show up in different ways during a physical exam. The ligaments that bind the vertebrae together and the muscles that stabilize and move the bones make up the broader intervertebral joint complex, which is the functional unit of the spine that allows you to move.

The facet surfaces have smooth linings made of cartilage, another type of connective tissue. In the very thin space between the cartilage linings is a lubricant, called synovial fluid, that allows the joint to move easily.

Causes of Back Pain

The back is a very complicated entity with lots of moving parts. When all the parts work in harmony, the back functions like a spectacular machine. But with so many pieces, there are many places where the machine can break down, resulting in dysfunction and pain.

The vast majority of lower back pain (about 98 percent of cases) is mechanical, or caused by physical stress and subsequent breakdown in your body.

The most common mechanical conditions include:

Spondylosis. This condition is basically long-term wear and tear. Over time, parts of your intervertebral joint can degenerate, which results in back pain. Because of the long-term nature of spondylosis, it's most common in the older population.

Stenosis. When the intervertebral joint breaks down, the body will often try to compensate by depositing more bone. This may narrow the space where the nerves exit, called the intervertebral foramen, or even the spinal canal itself. This narrowing puts pressure on the spinal nerves, which leads to pain.

Bulging and herniated discs. Discs consist of two parts: the gelatinous inner nucleus pulposis and the tough outer annulus fibrosus. With long-term mechanical stress, the nucleus may start to break through the inner fibers of the annulus. The first thing that may subsequently occur is a bulging at the back of the disc. Over time, the nucleus can break through (or herniate) the outer fibers of

Serious Conditions

While most back pain has mechanical causes and is the result of long-term stress and strain on the soft tissue structures, occasionally the underlying cause is a serious condition that requires medical attention. In these rare situations, the pain can develop slowly or suddenly.

Slower-building cases may be mistaken for standard back pain. However, the pain may be an indication of a growing bone tumor, either benign or cancerous, putting increased pressure on the nerves in the bone. That pain should feel different than traditional lower back pain. While movement generally triggers mechanical back pain, it won't affect pain from a bone tumor. Pain from a tumor may also feel worse at night and better during the day (when there are more distractions), whereas mechanical back pain is more persistent. If you suspect your slow, gradual back pain might be the result of a tumor, an X-ray or MRI should provide an initial diagnosis and a biopsy can confirm it.

Slow-developing back pain can also stem from a kidney infection (pyelonephritis), which results from an untreated bacterial infection moving up from the bladder. Other infections are also possible culprits behind slow-developing back pain, such as an infection in a vertebra (osteomyelitis) or in spinal discs (discitis). Lower back pain that results from an infection may also be accompanied by other symptoms, including fever, nausea, and a general sense of feeling sick. If you suspect your slow, gradual back pain might be the result of an infection, blood work and ultrasound imaging can provide a diagnosis, and a high dosage of antibiotics generally works as a treatment.

Lower back pain that comes on suddenly and sharply and doesn't go away warrants an immediate trip to the emergency room. It could be the result of kidney stones or a ruptured aortic aneurysm, both of which can be life-threatening and require immediate treatment.

the annulus. In both cases, the bulge or herniation can create pressure on the spinal nerve root as it exits. This pressure can cause localized lower back pain but also pain that radiates into the thigh and leg or neurological symptoms like decreased reflexes, altered sensations, and muscle weakness.

Sciatica. The sciatic nerve is made up of five nerve roots that exit the lumbar spine and sacrum. It's the largest nerve in the body and it's responsible for sensation and motor function from your hips all the way down to your toes. When any of the nerve roots are irritated, you may experience pain, numbness, or weakness that radiates into your thighs and legs. This irritating pressure is most often the result of a bulging or herniated disc, which is why sciatica can be a more advanced symptom of those conditions.

Piriformis syndrome. The piriformis muscle attaches to the sacrum and the hip. The sciatic nerve runs under this muscle. Excessive tension of the piriformis can put irritating pressure on the sciatic nerve that causes radiating pain down the leg, mimicking the symptoms of sciatica.

Sprain or strain. A sprain is an injury to the ligament fibers, and a strain is an injury to the muscle fibers. Ligaments are made of collagen-dense connective tissue fibers, whereas muscles are made of contracting fibers. The severity of a sprain or strain is determined by the percentage of fibers that are torn. Muscles are rich in blood, so a strain will heal much more quickly than a sprain. Both sprains and strains can be caused by sudden mechanical stresses, like twisting your ankle or experiencing whiplash in a car accident.

Traumatic injuries. Every structure in the lower back is wired with nerves, so injury to any of them can cause pain. Your body's response to trauma is inflammation, or the release of biochemicals into the tissues. This inflammation irritates your nerves, which you feel as pain.

Some patients ask me if they have a pinched nerve. Many people believe a pinched nerve is a more serious condition than those in which the nerve is not being pinched. This is not true. Whenever you have pain, a nerve is being pinched (i.e. irritated). Nerves mediate pain. The question is not whether the person has a pinched nerve, but rather *where* the nerve is being pinched—the ligament, the muscle, the disc, the facet, or somewhere else? The real issues are the location of injury and the severity of the nerve irritation. These determinations can help guide treatment, whether on your own or with the assistance of a healing practitioner.

Emotions and Back Pain

The relationship between the mind and the body has been the subject of historical interest and a great deal of research. Most of us have experienced this connection. When something suddenly frightens you, you may lose your appetite because of the tension you feel in your gut. Getting ready for a blind date, your palms may get sweaty because you are nervous. When you're walking down the street at night alone and hear footsteps behind you, you feel the blood rush through your body and the hairs on your arms and neck stand up.

There may be a relationship between what goes on in your mind and what you feel in your back. When you experience stress, one of the primary responses is that your whole body tenses up. This is the fight-or-flight response, which can be traced back through the history of human evolution. When you perceive a threat, your body prepares to either confront the source or run from it. Your muscles tighten so they are primed to attack or escape.

This response is very helpful when you suddenly find yourself in a dangerous situation, but not many people experience life-or-death confrontations on a regular basis. Nonetheless, the fight-or-flight response is still triggered regularly. Imagine you find out on Thursday afternoon that your boss needs a report done by nine sharp the next morning. You don't have the necessary command of the material to do this work, and you are already feeling insecure in your position. The fight-or-flight response will be activated, but it will not help you finish the report.

If you have an underlying mechanical problem in your discs, muscles, or tendons, it may be exacerbated by the muscle tension that accompanies your fight-or-flight response. When this stress is sustained over a longer period of time, the tightened muscles become fatigued and weak, further compromising the integrity of your musculoskeletal system. In addition, chronic emotional stress can cause generalized inflammation that creates or contributes to your pain.

If emotional stress is one of the contributing causes of your pain, you can address it. When you feel the tension and pain increasing, take five conscious breaths. Focus on breathing in, then breathing out. If your mind wanders, return your concentration to your breath. This practice can help calm your nervous system and relax your body.

Although this breathing exercise might be a good short-term strategy, it's important to find activities to help relax your muscles on an ongoing basis. Perhaps you can start a simple meditation practice, such as sitting on a pillow for 10 minutes per day without any outside distractions. There is a movement called forest bathing that recognizes the health benefits of walking in the woods, breathing in the oxygen being released by the trees, and immersing yourself in the positive energy of the grove. You may find it more relaxing to listen to music, dance, or spend time at the beach.

If you aren't able to find an effective self-help strategy to relieve the emotional stress that may be contributing to your back pain, please seek professional support.

Risk Factors

Quite a few factors can elevate your risk for lower back pain. You can control many of them, but others may be beyond your reach. It is important to consider how to minimize or eliminate the risks when at all possible.

Fitness level. Your general fitness level is one of the most significant factors of overall health. Being in good cardio shape and maintaining lean body mass with solid core strength goes a long way toward preventing back pain.

Occupation. Another major factor of back pain is occupational risk. Almost every job poses potential problems. There are hazards for workers doing repetitive manual work as well as those sitting in front of computer screens all day. I treat many people with back pain who do both kinds of work.

The riskiest movement for people in physical jobs is bending forward from the torso (also known as the trunk), and it's even more dangerous if the bend is combined with a twist. This motion puts a lot of mechanical stress on the discs, which can lead to bulging. If there is already underlying wear and tear on the discs, the bending and/or twisting will worsen the damage and can turn a bulge into a herniation. The movement will also stress the other parts of the intervertebral joint complex, including the ligaments, muscles, and cartilage.

For office workers, sitting all day can be just as bad for the back as lifting cinder blocks. The more you sit, the more likely you are to start slouching.

Rounding your lower back is basically the same, from a mechanical perspective, as bending at the waist. In other words, sitting all day may seem less physically intense, but it's not all that different from doing repetitive manual labor. In both cases, you're putting excess pressure on your discs and other soft tissue structures of your back.

Obesity. The more weight you gain, the more work it takes to move your body. The added weight puts extra demand and strain on your back, which makes you more prone to injuries. But potential injuries are just part of the problem. A lesser-known reason for the increased lower-back risk with obesity is biochemical, not mechanical. Lean, healthy body fat is made up of small fat cells and anti-inflammatory immune cells. Obese body fat, on the other hand, is made of large, fat-crammed cells and pro-inflammatory immune cells. These obese fat cells release pro-inflammatory chemicals into your circulatory system, which can stimulate special nerve cells that transmit painful sensations.

Pregnancy. During pregnancy, a woman's center of gravity moves forward, and her body naturally adds extra weight. Both factors cause the back muscles to work harder and make it more difficult to move and simply stay upright. The extra weight adds stress to the supportive soft tissue structures of the back.

Age. Many people believe lower back pain mostly affects the older population, but that is not true. Over the past few decades, schools have placed increasingly physical demands on children, as early on as elementary school, to carry backpacks full of heavy books. As a result, it is not unusual in my practice to see 9- and 10-year-old children being treated for back pain.

Mental health. The relationship between mental health and lower back pain should not be minimized. If you already have a mechanical or structural imbalance that can potentially cause pain, added emotional stress can exacerbate the underlying problem. There is also clinical evidence of a potential relationship between depression and back pain. In these cases, antidepressants may be a helpful treatment option. (For more on the topic, see the discussion on page 12 on the connection between emotions and back pain.)

Genetics. Some people are genetically predisposed to experience back pain, so you can thank your parents for it. You may have inherited weaker disc tissue that makes it susceptible to herniation. Maybe you have tighter muscles that get in the way of proper joint function. Some people may even be born with malformed vertebral joints. Fortunately, a medical professional can take your genetic factors into consideration, treat your back pain, and get you on a path to relief.

CHAPTER 2

Diagnosis and Treatment

Most cases of lower back pain will resolve themselves on their own within a few weeks. If yours does not, however, it's a good idea to consult a health-care provider. A complete physical exam will help your practitioner figure out what type of care is appropriate and if you need to see other specialists for more diagnostic tests to rule out nonmechanical causes of your pain.

You may not realize it, but many experts start examining you from the moment they greet you. When I meet a new patient, I pay attention to all the little giveaways of back pain. How easily can you get out of your chair? Are you using the chair arms for support? Is your gait stiff and slow? Are you leaning to one side to avoid pain?

During the next stage of the exam, the practitioner reviews your medical history and asks questions. Do you need to stand because you feel pain when you're sitting? When did the pain begin? Was it sudden or did it come on gradually? Is it constant or on and off? What makes the pain worse? What relieves it? What is the quality of the pain—sharp, achy, burning, or dull? What time is the pain better or worse? Does pain radiate down your leg or into your front or back? Is this the first time you've had back pain? If not, when was the first time? How often do you have episodes of back pain? On a scale of 1 to 10, where would you rate your pain? What is your broader medical history? Have you dealt with cancer, heart disease, or any other conditions that could shed some light on your pain?

A thorough physical exam usually follows, which should include testing your range of motion, reflexes and dermatomes (for nervous system function), and muscle strength. A lower back pain expert, like a chiropractor, will use special palpation techniques to feel the motion of the joints of the lumbar spine and pelvis. They will also feel the muscles for tension and knots, also called trigger points.

Once the exam is done, the practitioner will be able to recommend an appropriate treatment for your specific case. This could involve treating you in their office or referring you for other diagnostic tests with another provider.

Testing Types

The majority of patients who come to my office with lower back pain can begin treatment without imaging or other advanced tests. But in some cases, more testing is necessary to properly identify the source of their pain. Here is a basic outline of what the tests are and in which situations they may be necessary.

X-ray. Although X-ray is the most common type of imaging, it cannot show soft tissues, such as discs, ligaments, and muscles, so it has limited value in diagnosing lower back pain cases. Most practitioners order X-rays only if the patient may have a tumor or a broken bone or isn't responding well to regular treatments. An X-ray will show decreased disc spaces, joint degeneration, abnormal spinal curvatures, and underlying joint anomalies like forward slippage of vertebrae (spondylolisthesis) or malformed facets (tropism).

Imaging: When to Use It, When to Avoid It

Medical imaging and blood tests can be very useful in arriving at a definitive diagnosis. If you go to the doctor with lower back pain and all evidence suggests the cause of the pain is mechanical, I do not recommend taking X-rays immediately. In practice, X-rays should be taken only if there is suspicion of a tumor, a fracture, or an anomaly. Unfortunately, some practitioners, even chiropractors, routinely X-ray all their patients and use the findings as a therapeutic guide.

There are also economic and legal reasons that imaging may be overused. If a doctor has a financial interest in an X-ray or MRI machine, they will be more likely to recommend these tests. As a savvy patient, it's important for you to ask the uncomfortable questions about conflicts of interest before agreeing to imaging tests.

Some medical-legal issues may drive imaging recommendations. We live in a litigious era, so some doctors may order more tests than are clinically necessary in order to protect themselves from future lawsuits. Many would rather err in doing too much than what they may perceive, out of fear, as too little.

Sometimes, however, further diagnostic testing is absolutely necessary. If there is a chance your pain is not mechanical, it's important to determine the cause as quickly as possible so you can get the right treatment. If your pain is not improving with treatment, it is crucial to find out why so you can move on to more productive therapy.

Be sure to involve a trusted health-care provider when deciding whether to go forward with diagnostic testing. Trust is built on having a practitioner who listens and has the clinical skills to manage your care effectively.

MRI (magnetic resonance imaging). MRI, another common type of imaging, uses magnetic frequencies to show a detailed picture of the vertebrae and the soft tissue that surrounds and attaches to them. MRIs reveal inflammation, protruding and herniated discs, muscle and ligament tears, and more. A practitioner can use an MRI with the results of a physical exam to provide a more accurate diagnosis.

CAT/CT Scan (computer axial tomography). Prior to MRI, CAT scans (now more commonly called CT scans) were the image of choice. CT scans use X-ray technology to produce high-quality images of bone and soft tissue. Although an MRI is generally preferred because it creates a more detailed image, there are some practical reasons to opt for a CT. First, it can image the body much more quickly than an MRI. Second, because the CT uses X-ray, not magnets, it can be used with patients who have metallic medical devices in their bodies.

Myelography. With a myelogram, a contrast dye is injected into the spinal canal before an X-ray or CT scan to help image the spinal cord and other nearby structures. Myelography is useful when other imaging techniques have not revealed the cause of pain.

Discography. This method is used to determine whether the disc is the source of the back pain. Needles are pushed into the disc and small amounts of dye are injected while the procedure is guided by a continuous X-ray (fluoroscopy) and imaged by CT scan. This test is often used after other images, such as MRI, have failed to identify the cause of back pain.

Bone scan. A bone scan involves injecting small amounts of radioactive materials into the bone and reading the waves that are emitted. It is used to hunt down hard-to-detect problems in the bones.

Blood tests. Blood work is used when the cause of pain might be systemic, rather than mechanical. For example, specific blood markers can point to autoimmune-related conditions like psoriatic or rheumatoid arthritis.

EMG (electromyography). EMG is a diagnostic procedure in which stickers or needles are placed along an extremity to determine the conduction of signals along a spinal nerve. This test is often used in conjunction with visual imaging to confirm a nerve or muscle dysfunction diagnosis.

Treatment Options

Your treatment options generally depend on whether your condition is acute or chronic. It's best to take a methodical approach to treatment, starting with the most conservative, noninvasive procedures. If significant neurological symptoms, like leg numbness or pain, won't subside, it may be time to consider surgery.

If you have acute lower back pain, your medical doctor will most likely want to see if simple self-care treatments will make the pain will go away as quickly as it came on. They will likely recommend taking it easy on your back (no heavy lifting), incorporating a program of gentle stretching and exercise, applying ice compresses, and taking a nonsteroidal anti-inflammatory medication, a muscle relaxer, or a painkiller. Most acute lower back pain goes away after two to six weeks. Once the pain dissipates, you should start a preventive program like the ones covered in this book. Without such a program, your back pain is very likely to return.

If you have chronic lower back pain, your doctor may add physical therapy to your treatment regimen and prescribe a more powerful anti-inflammatory medication like prednisone, which is a steroid.

MEDICATIONS

One of the trickiest parts of treating chronic pain is that it can lead to people using over-the-counter and prescription medicines for a long period of time. Even if medications are prescribed and taken with good intention to promote healing and relieve pain, they carry their own sets of complications.

Opiates like Oxycontin, Norco, and Vicodin are commonly prescribed for acute and chronic pain. Unfortunately, opiates can be highly addictive, and if you take them over the long term, it can be difficult to wean yourself off them.

Ibuprofen and naproxen are commonly prescribed nonsteroidal anti-inflammatory medications. Although these medications are available without a prescription, chronic use can damage the kidneys, liver, and other parts of the gastrointestinal system.

Some everyday over-the-counter medications can be hazardous. For example, pregnant women shouldn't take ibuprofen or aspirin for pain, but they can take Tylenol (acetaminophen).

It is important to talk with your doctor before you begin taking medications for your lower back pain to understand both the short- and long-term risks.

NONINVASIVE ALTERNATIVES

There is an intermediate step between basic lower back pain treatments (like rest, medication, and time) and surgery, which is the most drastic option. Some noninvasive alternatives may help you find relief.

Chiropractic. Back pain is central to most chiropractic practices, including my own. The approach is the same regardless of whether you have acute or chronic pain. The chiropractor will examine you, determine what exercises and stretches you should be doing, and start you on these movements immediately. If your muscles are tight or spasming, soft tissue massage techniques can reduce the tension. If your spinal joints aren't moving because your muscles are tight and irritating your nerves, spinal manipulation can mobilize the area. After this treatment, your chiropractor may put an ice pack on your lower back to reduce any inflammation the treatment might have stirred up. The goal of a chiropractic treatment is to reduce your pain, of course, but also to provide you with the knowledge and tools you need to continue healing your back and prevent the pain from recurring.

Physical therapy. Physical therapists take a similar approach to chiropractors, but their training and expertise lies in rehab exercises. Many physical therapists work in a gym setting with weights, treadmills, stationary bikes, and mats. They are usually very hands-on, making sure their patients are doing the exercises with correct form to minimize the chances of injury.

Osteopathy. Osteopathic medicine confuses many people. In the late 1800s and early 1900s, osteopathy was very similar to chiropractic care. In fact, there is credible evidence that the founder of chiropractic, Daniel David Palmer, stole his ideas from Andrew Taylor Still, the founder of osteopathy. Originally, osteopathic treatment consisted of hands-on joint and muscle manipulation, much like chiropractic. Over time, however, the osteopathic field of practitioners, through their professional organization, made an agreement with their medical counterparts to get parity to become equal with medical doctors. Since that time, most osteopaths have gone into specialties, just like medical doctors, such as orthopedist, neurologist, and nephrologist. The only difference is that after their names the letters are DO (doctor of osteopathy) rather than MD (medical doctor). A small percentage of osteopaths still do hands-on work for back pain and other conditions. If you see an osteopath for your back pain treatment, make sure they specialize in the hands-on care that was an original part of the osteopathic approach.

Acupuncture. Acupuncture, which involves inserting needles at very specific points along the skin surface, is just one part of a much broader ancient system called Traditional Chinese Medicine (TCM). TCM also encompasses herbal medicine, exercise, meditation, and multiple deep tissue therapies. During episodes of back pain, acupuncture can help relax your muscles, reduce your inflammation and pain, and even soothe your anxiety.

Rolfing. A variety of soft tissue techniques focus on balancing the musculoskeletal system and reducing pain. One of the most well-known is Rolfing, or structural integration. Rolfing gets its unusual name from its creator, biochemist Ida Rolf, who developed the practice in the 1960s. Rolfing features a series of specific deep-tissue therapy sessions focused on the fascia, or the linings between the muscles. The sessions can be painful, as the practitioner is working to release the muscles so they can move more freely. When your muscles are free, your posture improves, which keeps you more balanced and helps you avoid pain.

Yoga. While yoga may sometimes be associated with designer workout apparel and classes that involve goats or paddleboards, this well-known exercise system is part of Ayurveda, a much broader ancient Indian medical system. Ayurveda includes nutritional, herbal, meditative, and medicinal components. Today, yoga has evolved into its own rehab exercise system, and yoga therapists can treat people for chronic lower back pain.

There are many more noninvasive back pain treatments, including Pilates, Feldenkrais, Alexander technique, Hellerwork, and spinal decompression. But the big question is, which methods are actually effective? One of the challenges in choosing a treatment is that the scientific evidence for all of them is highly inconclusive. Very little consensus exists, even among experts.

Practitioners definitely agree on one thing: If you have back pain, you should not stop moving. Years ago, many experts believed the best treatment for back pain was for the patient to lie down, be still, and let the back heal itself. The theory was that moving when in pain would cause even more damage.

We now know that movement is essential, both for healing back pain and for preventing recurrence. When you stop moving, your supportive muscles become weaker and put more stress into your joints, which slows the healing process. Any approach to treating back pain should have an active component. Passive therapies are treatments that are done *to* you, like spinal manipulation, massage therapy, ultrasound, electrical stimulation, or traction. Active therapies require your participation and amplify the positive effects of the passive therapy.

A variety of movement techniques, like Pilates and yoga, may be helpful in relieving your back pain. If you're dealing with chronic lower back pain, work with your Pilates, yoga, or other instructor in coordination with your health-care professional.

CONSIDERING SURGERY

If you've exhausted all conservative methods to treat your chronic lower back pain and you're showing specific neurological symptoms, like radiating leg pain or trouble with your reflexes, surgery might be an option.

Generally, before deciding on surgery, your doctor will refer you for an epidural injection into the area where they suspect your nerves are irritated. This steroid injection should reduce the inflammation that is putting pressure on the nerve and causing the symptoms. The treatment has two benefits: It's therapeutic, and it can help provide a clearer diagnosis of your problem. If your lower back pain or leg symptoms are relieved by the injection, you've confirmed the location and cause of the pain. Sometimes the epidural can resolve the pain altogether. If it doesn't or it gives you only short-term relief, you may be a candidate for surgery.

While surgery is sometimes necessary, you'll have to weigh the risks against the rewards. One of the challenges of surgery for lower back pain is that even with all the diagnostic tools and techniques available, it can still be difficult to identify the precise cause of your pain. A skilled and ethical surgeon will proceed only when that cause is clear.

Some of the procedures performed for lower back pain include:

Spinal fusion. This procedure is most common. Either part or all of a spinal disc is removed (discectomy or microdiscectomy), and the vertebrae above and below are attached to each other to allow space for a compressed nerve to exit the spinal canal without being irritated. (Sometimes a microdiscectomy may take care of the problem and a fusion is not necessary.)

Laminectomy. This procedure involves removing the back part of the vertebrae (lamina) to relieve pressure on the exiting spinal nerve. Removal of the bone can make that segment of the spine unstable, however, so you may need a spinal fusion in the future. There is also an option to have an interlaminar implant to replace the bone that is removed. This procedure can help stabilize the area so you'll be less likely to need fusion surgery later on.

Disc replacement. In this procedure, the damaged disc is removed and an artificial one replaces it, and a fusion is not necessary. The intervertebral joint can maintain more normal motion, decreasing the chance of new disc problems developing in the joints above or below.

When spinal surgery is successful, it can seem like a miracle. Patients often report an almost immediate reduction of symptoms, but sometimes relief is only temporary or the symptoms don't resolve at all. It's not unusual after a successful fusion for segments near the treated area to break down and require additional surgery. You lose some mobility with spinal fusion, which puts more stress on the other spinal segments.

Potential negative side effects of surgery include a bad reaction to the general anesthesia, infection, or nerve damage that can lead to paralysis, sexual dysfunction, or loss of bladder or bowel control. While such side effects rarely occur, it is important that you are fully informed about their possibility. Given the very real risks associated with surgery, it's crucial to find a skilled surgeon who can answer all your questions.

The Truth about Prevention

Recurring back pain is usually caused by a series of problematic movements and postures at work and at home. If you want to prevent back pain from occurring or returning, it's important to understand what you're doing wrong and make the necessary corrections.

At work, common causes of back pain are sitting too much and repetitive and awkward lifting. Keep these tips in mind to protect yourself.

Set up an ergonomic workstation. If you're one of the 86 percent of Americans who sits at a desk all day, it's important to set up your workstation properly. The center of your computer monitor should be at eye level and directly in front of you. If you prevent sustained looking up or down, left or right, you minimize the chances of back strain and pain. Make sure you have a good chair that's at the correct height and provides good lower back support. Your feet should rest flat on the floor.

Stand up and stretch. Take a few minutes to stand up at least every 45 minutes to do some basic stretches, like shoulder rolls and chest pull backs. Over the course of the day, people tend to slouch in their chairs (which is why you need good lumbar support), so doing some gentle backbends will help relieve the tension that has built up in your lower back muscles.

Practice deep breathing. Incorporating deep breathing will help relax your entire body and bring your shoulders back to improve your posture and reduce strain.

Lift properly. If you do physical work that involves lifting, make sure you understand the basics of proper form. One of the most stressful movements for the lower back is bending at the waist to lift a load. Even worse is combining that forward bend with a twist, which puts a tremendous amount of strain on the soft tissue structures of the lower back, especially the discs. When you're lifting an object, face it, bend at your knees, bring the object as close to your body as possible, and lift from your knees with your lower back straight. The difference between lifting safely or dangerously is being mindful of good form and taking two or three seconds to do it correctly. When you are working quickly and feeling rushed, you can forget to take care of how you engage your body.

Use back support. Many warehouse and factory workers wear lower back support belts, but you should use one only if you have active lower back pain. The belt provides external support to the postural muscles of the lower back and allows them to rest and heal. If you are not in pain, however, and wear the belt to prevent a lower back injury, you may actually cause more damage. Wearing the support all day can cause the muscles to weaken and make them *more* susceptible to injury. I've had patients who wear a lower back support at work and get hurt at home mowing the lawn or lifting their baby.

You can do a lot to ease your lower back pain and speed up your healing process. An exercise program that stretches and strengthens your back can help heal acute back pain and prevent repeat episodes in the future. The remainder of this book gives you the tools to build a stronger back. While exercise can be hard work, it can also be fun. Enjoy the process!

CHAPTER 3

Habits for a Healthy Back

This book is for everyone, not just those who have lower back pain and are ready to start a stretching and exercise program. If you have never been (or aren't currently) in pain, you can still do many things to prevent lower back issues from developing or returning. On the other end of the spectrum, if you're experiencing so much pain that even the easy strengthening program in this book seems too intense, you can do other activities to start on the road to recovery. Whatever your current situation, you'll reap great benefits from adopting the habits in this chapter.

Research has shown that movement is essential for healing. Today, bed rest is rarely prescribed to treat back pain. Even if you're in significant pain, you should get moving as soon as possible—under the guidance of a trained professional, if necessary.

In addition to movement, it's important to focus on your posture. Poor lifting techniques or slouching at your desk will put a lot of strain on the structures of your lower back.

The spine is a beautifully engineered system with four different curves. The neck curves forward (called a lordosis), the middle back curves backward (called a kyphosis), the lower back again curves forward, and the sacrum and coccyx curve backward. The spine is perfectly designed to withstand the effects of gravity and normal forces of everyday life, but its effectiveness rests on the integrity of your back muscles, tendons, ligaments, and discs. The remainder of this book focuses on how to maintain your back integrity.

One general rule before we dive in: If your lower back pain is accompanied by radiating leg pain, stop any movement that exacerbates the leg pain. A movement that causes leg pain is a signal that a spinal nerve is being irritated and the exercise is more harmful than helpful. On the other hand, a movement that reduces leg pain but increases back pain is generally viewed in a positive light. But if your lower back pain is accompanied by radiating back pain, a trained health-care practitioner should supervise your exercise program.

The Cardio Component

Three activities comprise what I call the three pillars of spinal health: cardio, stretching, and core strengthening. This section addresses all three, starting with cardio.

You may be wondering what so many of my patients have asked me: "Why cardio? My back hurts."

It's a fair question, because on the surface it's hard to see a connection between doing cardio exercise and a having healthy back. But every structure in your body depends on healthy circulation. Your body is a complex system of moving parts, each of which is powered by energy. The circulatory system delivers that energy: Nutrients are delivered from the digestive system and oxygen through the respiratory system. The more efficient your blood supply, the better your muscles will function.

Blood also carries healing chemicals to injured tissues, such as muscles, tendons, ligaments, and discs. Your body then responds automatically, on a bio-chemical level, to heal itself. And because you're constantly doing damage to your tissues with physical activity and less-than-perfect posture, increased blood flow will speed up the healing process. You may not even be aware of the micro injuries present throughout your body, but a constant cycle of healing is taking place.

When energy is produced, so is waste. Another function of the blood vessels is to transport the waste products your soft tissue naturally generates. Muscle contractions lead to buildup of lactic acid, pyruvic acid, and hyaluronic acid, and in healthy muscles, the small blood vessels carry this waste away and filter it out through the kidneys.

But if your blood is not flowing smoothly, acids can build up in the muscles, irritating nerves, causing pain, and leading to tightness and small areas of fibrous nodules you probably know as knots.

A muscle injury (strain) takes much less time to heal than a ligament injury (sprain) because the blood supply in a muscle is much richer than in a ligament. But the more you move your body, the more your blood will move, and the healthier your back will be.

Cardio exercise can be intimidating, especially if it's not a regular part of your daily activities. If you're new to it, start with gentle low-impact movement. This habit will help you start to build up your endurance and maintain a healthy weight. You don't need to compete in a triathlon; you just need to be up and moving around as best you can.

Most health-care professionals recommend doing 20 to 30 minutes of cardio exercise three or four times a week. Choose activities that burn calories and don't put too much stress on your joints.

Hiking is my favorite form of cardio. I'm very fortunate to live in a place that has beautiful trees and plenty of big hills. When I want to exercise, I walk out my door, put on my headphones, and make a right turn. Exercise not only raises your heart rate, but also relaxes your mind. As blood flows, your muscles get stronger and so does your brain. The fresh, healthy air keeps the oxygen flowing through your lungs and invigorates the rest of your body.

It's important to find an activity that works for you so you will stick with it. Maybe you love to swim and have access to a pool or lake. You might live in a dense city and find having a stationary bike in your apartment is the best way to go. These bikes are now quite sophisticated, with programs to make you feel like you are riding along the California coastline or through quaint towns in the south of France. You can even remotely connect to classes and have a live instructor coach you. If you enjoy going to the gym, you can use an elliptical trainer or a rowing machine. If you loathe jogging and hate waking up early, don't declare you're going to go for a run every morning at dawn.

When you're doing cardio outdoors, be mindful of your surroundings. Keep an eye out for uneven surfaces where you might twist an ankle or throw your body out of alignment. Wear supportive and comfortable shoes made for the activity you're doing. When I'm hiking on rocky trails, I wear my hiking boots. It pains me to see people on the same rough trails in regular sneakers or, even worse, flip-flops! (I almost feel like I should hand them my business card, because I know they'll need me in the future.)

If you want to hike steep trails but you're nervous about falling, use trekking poles. Don't be embarrassed! The poles assist greatly with balance and stability and help minimize the risk of injury.

Before you go from a low-impact cardio workout to a rigorous one, remember to check in with your physician on your condition and appropriate activity levels. You want to rule out any health risks before you level up.

Applied Mechanics

Another important key to maintaining a healthy back is paying attention to your body mechanics and posture when you're standing, sitting, and moving.

As you move through the world, the mechanical forces on your body are constantly changing. Your back is well designed to withstand normal stresses, but a lot of activities that seem innocent are actually quite stressful and potentially damaging to your back. Driving, sitting at a desk, playing with your kids, grand-kids, or dog, doing the laundry, carrying the groceries, and even reading in bed can put your back in compromising positions. These everyday actions gener-ally don't cause immediate pain, however, which leads many people to develop unhealthy habits.

There are two types of back injuries:

Sudden. This type of pain is the result of a specific incident. For example, you walk across the street and get hit by a car (although let's hope that never hap-pens). In this case, it is easy to identify when your back pain started.

Gradual. This type of pain is more typical. For example, you work as a hairstylist, which involves holding up your arms for hours each day and bending forward a great deal. These movements transfer mechanical stress into all the soft tissue structures of your upper and lower back. Your muscles slowly get tighter. You might feel some soreness as pain-sensitive nerve endings are stimulated. Then, one morning, you are blow-drying your hair after a shower and suddenly you can't move your neck. Your muscles are spasming and you have sharp pain going from the base of your skull to your shoulder blade. The motion of drying your hair did not cause the problem; it was just (please pardon or deeply appreciate this pun) the straw that broke the camel's back. Over time, small movements and habits can cause serious back problems.

So much of prevention is really awareness. It's critical to be mindful of damaging movements and postures and understand some basic biomechanics.

Standing with good posture requires the coordination of all your muscles, ligaments, and discs. When they're all properly balanced, the mechanical stresses are distributed properly so none of the soft tissue structures are bearing an unequal amount of the load. The proper position is called neutral posture, described by the Office of Environment, Health and Safety at the University of California, San Francisco, as "a position of ease for the body to maintain for a prolonged period of time; a position that supports the natural curves of the spine and maintains your body in good alignment; [and] a position of ease for the body to sustain with minimal effort." Once you deviate from that balanced posture, strain builds and you risk injury.

Remember, the primary problematic movement for the lower back is bending forward at the waist. The worst is bending forward while twisting. With that in mind, let's look at some day-to-day scenarios that can cause problems and explore how you can minimize the dangers.

Doing laundry. When you do laundry, chances are you're bending down to load the machine, move clothes from the washer to the dryer, and fold dry clothes. When you're folding, a big load can keep you bent over for 10 to 15 minutes, long enough to feel your lower back straining. To avoid that strain, try folding on a higher surface or sitting while you fold. At the very least, fold for a few minutes and then do some backbends, which will put some healthy opposite motion into your lumbar spine.

Sitting on the couch. When you're sitting on a couch or a soft chair, you may feel like you're sinking into it. You are, and it's causing your lower back to round.

This movement is the mechanical equivalent of bending forward at the waist. It's best to avoid really soft seats altogether, especially if you're having lower back pain. But if you must sit on one, put a small pillow behind your lower back. It will passively force you into the correct posture. Choose a chair with arms, whenever possible, so you can push yourself from sitting to standing using your arm muscles, rather than your back.

Wearing high heels. Heels force your lower back into a sustained, exaggerated arching (hyperextension), which can cause irritation on the back part, or facets, of your intervertebral joints. While you may enjoy the aesthetic effect of high heels, it is best to avoid them. If you have a rare situation where you must wear them, try to minimize the duration.

Sleeping. You don't want to damage your back while you sleep, so the best preventive measure is to use lots of pillows. If you're a back sleeper, put one or two pillows under your knees. If you're a side sleeper, put them between your knees. If you're a stomach sleeper, put them under your stomach.

Once you understand these healthy principles, you can apply them to any new situations you may encounter. It's all about minimizing the mechanical stresses. The closer you can get to normal posture when you're sitting, standing, or lying down, the happier your back will be.

HOW TO SIT AT A DESK

Because my practice is in San Francisco, one of the tech centers of the world, I treat a lot of people who spend their days (and often nights) sitting in front of a computer. If you're at a desk, whether for a long day of work or just a few hours, it's important to sit in the correct position. Fortunately, an ergonomic revolution in recent years has created quite a few options for minimizing the mechanical stress of prolonged sitting. Here's what you'll need for your workstation.

Ergonomic chair. When you're choosing a chair, keep in mind a few important features. You should be able to move the chair up and down so you can lock it at a height where your feet rest flat on the floor. If the height of your desk makes that impossible, use a footstool. The seat of the chair, also called the pan, should clear your legs below the knee. Finally, you must have good lumbar support. In the same way sitting on a soft couch can round the lower back, extended periods in your work chair can do the same. Good lower back support will keep your lumbar spine in its correct curved position and enable you to remain upright.

I'd like to clear up a few misunderstandings about sitting posture. Some people claim the hip angle, where the thigh meets the pelvis, should be 90 degrees. I have even seen some recommendations that the knees should be slightly higher than the hips. This is incorrect. The goal is to maintain the normal curves of the spine. As you raise your knees, you flatten the lumbar curve, as though you were sitting in a soft chair. The ideal hip angle is pointed down, closer to 100 to 130 degrees. Consider looking into an ergonomic chair with a cutout for your hips so you can maintain that high hip angle while you sit upright with good lumbar support and you don't risk sliding out of your chair.

Another common problem is when people don't lock the back rests of their chairs so they can rock back and forth throughout the day. While you may get some relief by going from upright to semi-reclined, when you get into upright

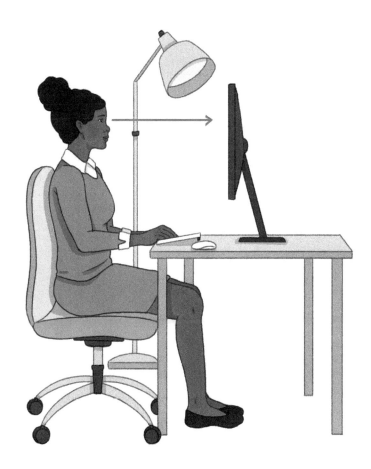

posture, your lower back support is lost unless you continuously lock and unlock the seat back.

When you're in a healthy, neutral posture, whether sitting or standing, not only will your back feel better, but your mind will also have more clarity and you'll be more efficient.

Sit/stand desk. Evolution did not build us to sit all day. We were born to move. The introduction of the sit/stand desk has helped with promoting movement. The ability to move from sitting to standing and back to sitting enables you to avoid the sustained mechanical stress of either position all day long.

Sit/stand desks come in various forms. Motorized electric desks with control switches allow you to set the heights for various tasks. Manual desks controlled by a hydraulic handle allow you to change the desk height quickly. Desktop converters transform your regular desk into a sit/stand model.

When you're choosing a desk, make sure you pick one you will use over the long term. I often compare sit/stand desks to gym memberships. Many of us signed up at a health club and spent the first month going five days each week. A few months later, we realize we haven't been there for weeks. Similarly, some people use the sit/stand function initially and then just keep it locked in one position, never to be moved again.

The ideal ratio of sitting to standing during the day goes from 1:1 to 1:3. You should spend anywhere from half the day standing to three-quarters of the day standing. Whatever ratio you choose, make sure to go back and forth between standing and sitting, changing positions anywhere from once every hour to once every three hours.

One final note: The key to a healthy back is healthy movement. Even if you have the best ergonomic chair in the world, if you sit in that chair for three hours without getting up, you will stress the structures of your back and set yourself up for injury. Try standing up, walking for a few minutes, rolling your shoulders, drinking some water, and taking deep breaths.

A Word on Weight and Nutrition

What if it is difficult to move? If your energy is low? If it just feels tough to get up off your chair or your couch? If you carry excess weight, it can impact your lower back pain both mechanically and biochemically.

But what is excess weight? The main tool used to classify weight is the body mass index, or BMI. It's calculated by dividing your weight in kilograms by the square of your height in meters. The number is a percentage, which falls into a category: underweight, healthy weight, overweight, or obese. BMI is an imperfect metric, as there are a variety of reasons people may fall into a BMI category that appears to be unhealthy. For example, a marathon runner may seem underweight and a football player with single-digit body fat but lots of muscle may show up as overweight. As a general rule, people who fall into the category of obese (a BMI greater than 30) are at risk for a variety of metabolic disorders, including diabetes and heart disease.

It's also more likely that people with a high BMI that registers as overweight or obese will have back pain. There are several reasons for this correlation:

- As the center of gravity moves forward because of increased belly fat, it places extra mechanical stress on the muscles and joints of the back. Men in particular are likely to carry more of their excess weight around their midsection.

- The increased weight leads to more forces compressing the intervertebral joint complex.

- With increased weight, and especially obesity, a person is less likely to get the exercise they need to support a healthy back.

- People who are overweight, especially the elderly, have a greater chance of injuring themselves in a fall.

- Healing can be slower because of an overtaxed circulatory system and increased inflammation.

Because there is a clear relationship between back pain and weight gain, the best approach to reducing weight-related back pain is to work on losing weight.

The healthiest way to simultaneously lose weight and reduce low-level inflammation (which can cause pain and prevent healing) is to eat an anti-inflammatory diet. Avoid foods like refined sugars, refined grains, trans fats, and omega-6 seed oils (including corn, safflower, and peanut). Replace them with healthy anti-inflammatory alternatives, such as lean meats, wild-caught fish, vegetables, roots, nuts, spices, olive oil, red wine, and dark chocolate. (Of course, even if you're eating healthy foods, consuming too many calories will keep the weight on, and your healthy diet will lead to inflammation.)

You can also help reduce inflammation and promote healthy tissue growth with supplements, including magnesium, vitamin D, and omega-3 fatty acids from fish oil. Ginger and turmeric are natural anti-inflammatories.

Finally, intermittent fasting can speed up weight loss and reduce inflammation. Intermittent fasting involves going at least 13 hours between the end of your eating on one day and the start of your eating the next day. For example, if you finish dinner at 7:00 p.m., you don't eat until 8:00 a.m. the following day. Over time, you can increase the number of fasting hours. Try it, and watch the pounds come off and your energy improve. However, I recommend speaking to your health-care provider about whether intermittent fasting is right for you before starting a self-directed program. You want to be sure you have no particular health risks, such as fainting or losing an unhealthy amount of weight.

PART II

THE BACK PAIN ACTION PLAN

T he goal of developing your exercise program is to help you build strong, flexible muscles that will be less prone to injury. Healthy muscles help support healthy joints.

If you're experiencing acute back pain, your goal is to resume normal activities as soon as possible. If you suffer from chronic back pain, you should work with a physician to come up with goals and milestones for a stretching and strengthening program.

In either case, pain relief is always a top priority. Most people show up in my office in pain and want to get rid of it immediately, but resolving symptoms isn't enough. It's equally important, especially for a long, pain-free life, to get to the root causes of the symptoms. Once you've determined the pain's origin, you can develop an appropriate action plan.

In the majority of cases, the problems are mechanical. You're in pain because your lower back muscles are in spasm, but the root cause might be sitting on your couch with your laptop for five hours a day. Work with your practitioner on ways to improve your posture (such as putting a small pillow under your lower back), incorporate more stretching breaks, improve nutrition and lose weight, and make your workspace more ergonomic.

After you've made day-to-day and lifestyle changes, it's time to move on to a stretching and strengthening program. A good program is essential for both acute and chronic lower back pain, even after you're symptom-free.

CHAPTER 4

Workout Programs

The "core" refers to the muscles of your trunk and extremities. Core strength is at the, well, core of a lower back strengthening program.

Core strength is built through balance and coordinated use of your muscles. The more years I practice, the more I see that so many of the mechanical problems we experience—not just lower back pain—come from the core.

You might notice that after you've wrapped up a rigorous ab workout, you stand up straighter, even though you didn't work directly on the upper back muscles responsible for your posture. That's because of the various mechanical and neurological connections between the core and the trunk above it.

> **Remember the golden rule of any exercise program:** If it causes you pain, stop! Exercise is not meant to hurt you. There are times, however, especially if you're dealing with chronic pain, that you need to push through a bit of discomfort as part of the healing process. Make sure you're working under the supervision of a health-care practitioner like a physical therapist or chiropractor.

Let's dive into a series of stretches and exercises designed to give you the physical support you need to have a healthy, pain-free back, now and in the future.

Action Plan Workouts

As I mentioned earlier, the three pillars of spinal health are cardio, stretching, and core strengthening. I'm going to start you off with stretching and cardio, but the ultimate goal is to combine all three. Over time, you'll want to move away from thinking about the pillars separately and recognize how they all work together as an integrated whole. The goal is stability, which means strength, flexibility, and balance.

I've put together four-week stretching, cardio, and strengthening programs at four levels: gentle, easy, medium, and advanced.

Start with the gentle program if you haven't exercised for a while. It's a great first step, and as you start stretching and getting your body moving, your goal will be to move up to the next level. The same goal applies if you start on the easy or medium program: Look at it as your starting point, not your ending point. Move up when you're ready to take on the added challenge and make even better progress on healing your back.

Of course, if any of the stretches cause you pain in your back or elsewhere, stop. Take the rest of the day off, examine your exercise form, and try again tomorrow, using half the recommended intensity.

Finally, let's address the elephant in the room: You may find stretching boring. Perhaps you'd rather head straight for the elliptical or the weight stacks. Once your workout is over, you prefer to shower and get on with your day, instead of stretching to cool down. But if your muscles aren't stretching, they will restrict the motion of all the joints up the kinetic chain. So even if you find stretching tedious, make the conscious, mindful choice to do it anyway. Your back will thank you.

GENTLE

The gentle program starts off with two weeks of light cardio to get your body moving. The next two weeks incorporate some stretches combined with more cardio.

When it comes to cardio choices, it's best to start with a low-intensity exercise, like taking a brisk walk on level ground or riding a stationary bike. There's no need to attempt the 400-meter hurdles on day one. If you are a senior, you can even do stretches in a chair.

	WEEK 1	WEEK 2	WEEK 3	WEEK 4
MONDAY	Cardio of choice (10–15 minutes)	Cardio of choice (10–15 minutes)	Cardio of choice (15 minutes)	Cardio of choice (15 minutes)
TUESDAY			1 or 2 stretches	3 or 4 stretches
WEDNESDAY	Cardio of choice (10–15 minutes)	Cardio of choice (10–15 minutes)	Cardio of choice (15 minutes)	Cardio of choice (15 minutes)
THURSDAY			1 or 2 stretches	3 or 4 stretches
FRIDAY	Cardio of choice (10–15 minutes)	Cardio of choice (10–15 minutes)	Cardio of choice (15 minutes)	Cardio of choice (15 minutes)
SATURDAY			1 or 2 stretches	3 or 4 stretches
SUNDAY		Cardio of choice (10–15 minutes)		Cardio of choice (15 minutes)

EASY

At this level, you crank up the cardio and do more stretches more regularly. If you're progressing up from the gentle program, the fourth week of that program featured four days of cardio. Let's stay with that through this month. If you can, pick up the pace (walk a little faster or bike a little harder) and push the duration up to 20 to 25 minutes.

	WEEK 1	WEEK 2	WEEK 3	WEEK 4
MONDAY	Cardio of choice (15–20 minutes)	Cardio of choice (15–20 minutes)	Cardio of choice (15–20 minutes)	Cardio of choice (15–20 minutes)
TUESDAY	4 or 5 stretches 1 or 2 easy exercises	4 or 5 stretches 1 or 2 easy exercises	5 or 6 stretches 3 or 4 easy exercises	5 or 6 stretches 2 easy exercises 2 medium exercises
WEDNESDAY	Cardio of choice (15–20 minutes)	Cardio of choice (15–20 minutes)	Cardio of choice (15–20 minutes)	Cardio of choice (15–20 minutes)
THURSDAY	4 or 5 stretches 1 or 2 easy exercises	4 or 5 stretches 1 or 2 easy exercises	5 or 6 stretches 3 or 4 easy exercises	5 or 6 stretches 2 easy exercises 2 medium exercises
FRIDAY	Cardio of choice (15–20 minutes)	Cardio of choice (15–20 minutes)	Cardio of choice (15–20 minutes)	Cardio of choice (15–20 minutes)
SATURDAY	4 or 5 stretches 1 or 2 easy exercises	4 or 5 stretches 1 or 2 easy exercises	5 or 6 stretches 3 or 4 easy exercises	5 or 6 stretches 2 easy exercises 2 medium exercises
SUNDAY	Cardio of choice (15–20 minutes)	Cardio of choice (15–20 minutes)	Cardio of choice (15–20 minutes)	Cardio of choice (15–20 minutes)

MEDIUM

The medium program increases the cardio up to 25 minutes, if that feels comfortable. I also recommend upping the intensity a bit. For example, if you've been taking brisk walks, find a hilly area and try to walk up hills at your previous pace. The medium program also mixes in even more stretches than the easy program and introduces supplemental equipment to augment your workout.

	WEEK 1	WEEK 2	WEEK 3	WEEK 4
MONDAY	Cardio of choice (20–25 minutes)	Cardio of choice (20–25 minutes)	Cardio of choice (20–25 minutes)	Cardio of choice (20–25 minutes)
TUESDAY	7 or 8 stretches 3 or 4 medium exercises	7 or 8 stretches 3 or 4 medium exercises	7 or 8 stretches 4 or 5 medium exercises	7 or 8 stretches 4 or 5 medium exercises
WEDNESDAY	Cardio of choice (20–25 minutes)	Cardio of choice (20–25 minutes)	Cardio of choice (20–25 minutes)	Cardio of choice (20–25 minutes)
THURSDAY	7 or 8 stretches 3 or 4 medium exercises	7 or 8 stretches 3 or 4 medium exercises	7 or 8 stretches 4 or 5 medium exercises	7 or 8 stretches 4 or 5 medium exercises
FRIDAY	Cardio of choice (20–25 minutes)	Cardio of choice (20–25 minutes)	Cardio of choice (20–25 minutes)	Cardio of choice (20–25 minutes)
SATURDAY	7 or 8 stretches 3 or 4 medium exercises	7 or 8 stretches 3 or 4 medium exercises	7 or 8 stretches 4 or 5 medium exercises	7 or 8 stretches 4 or 5 medium exercises
SUNDAY	Cardio of choice (20–25 minutes)	Cardio of choice (20–25 minutes)	Cardio of choice (20–25 minutes)	Cardio of choice (20–25 minutes)

ADVANCED

In the advanced level, it's important to push the pace of your cardio even more. Walk faster, bike harder, or incorporate more intense options like an elliptical machine. If you can push your total exercise time to 30 minutes, great. The advanced level also features more challenging exercises.

	WEEK 1	WEEK 2	WEEK 3	WEEK 4
MONDAY	Cardio of choice (20–30 minutes)	Cardio of choice (20–30 minutes)	Cardio of choice (20–30 minutes)	Cardio of choice (20–30 minutes)
TUESDAY	7 or 8 stretches 4 medium and 1 advanced exercises	7 or 8 stretches 3 medium and 2 advanced exercises	7 or 8 stretches 3 medium and 3 advanced exercises	7 or 8 stretches 2 medium and 4 advanced exercises
WEDNESDAY	Cardio of choice (20–30 minutes)	Cardio of choice (20–30 minutes)	Cardio of choice (20–30 minutes)	Cardio of choice (20–30 minutes)
THURSDAY	7 or 8 stretches 4 medium and 1 advanced exercises	7 or 8 stretches 3 medium and 2 advanced exercises	7 or 8 stretches 3 medium and 3 advanced exercises	7 or 8 stretches 2 medium and 4 advanced exercises
FRIDAY	Cardio of choice (20–30 minutes)	Cardio of choice (20–30 minutes)	Cardio of choice (20–30 minutes)	Cardio of choice (20–30 minutes)
SATURDAY	7 or 8 stretches 4 medium and 1 advanced exercises	7 or 8 stretches 3 medium and 2 advanced exercises	7 or 8 stretches 3 medium and 3 advanced exercises	7 or 8 stretches 2 medium and 4 advanced exercises
SUNDAY	Cardio of choice (20–30 minutes)	Cardio of choice (20–30 minutes)	Cardio of choice (20–30 minutes)	Cardio of choice (20–30 minutes)

The next chapter covers the stretches you can use at every level of the programs.

CHAPTER 5

Stretching

PIGEON GLUTE STRETCH 54

TFL WALL STRETCH 56

TFL FOAM ROLLING 58

PSOAS DOORWAY STRETCH 60

HAMSTRING DOORWAY STRETCH 62

STANDING QUADRICEPS STRETCH 64

BUTTERFLY ADDUCTORS STRETCH 66

LYING LEG REST PIRIFORMIS STRETCH 68

Stretching is vital to maintaining healthy movement. When you stop moving, your body begins to break down.

When I was 12 years old, I was playing baseball and the catcher tagged me hard on my side as I slid into home plate. (I still scored the run.) We quickly realized my kidney was damaged and I had to spend a week in a hospital bed. When I got out of bed after being immobilized, I couldn't walk. My muscles had atrophied, my joints had tightened up, and my father had to hold me up. I was young and healthy, so I bounced back quickly, but it was an early lesson on why movement is essential to living a healthy, functional life. And if that can happen to a 12-year-old after just one week of inactivity, imagine the effects on an older person or someone who has been inactive for a longer period of time.

When your intervertebral joints lose their mobility, they rapidly stiffen up. The cartilage depends on movement to pump in nutrients from the blood that help maintain healthy lubrication. When the joints stop moving or barely move, the surfaces become dry, ligaments that stabilize the joints tighten, and you lose your normal range of motion.

But the body, in its infinite wisdom, will often compensate for the lost motion by enabling the joints above or below the stuck (or hypomobile) segment to increase their motion. As a result, you end up with both hypomobile and hyper-mobile joints, and none of the joints function optimally. Over time, this joint dysfunction can lead to back pain.

Joint degeneration can lead to conditions like osteoarthritis, or inflammation of the joints. In addition, the loss of joint mobility will put more mechanical pressure on the discs and make it increasingly difficult to maintain proper posture. And on top of that, less flexible muscles can increase your chances of strains and sprains.

It is important to stretch to maintain mobility, to keep your joints healthy and doing their proper jobs, to prevent injuries, and to avoid developing conditions that can cause short- and long-term back pain.

There are a variety of different stretching methods, but the most common is static stretching, when you bring a muscle to the end of its range of motion and hold the position for 20 to 30 seconds or more.

Other stretching methods can also be very effective. Some may require assistance, whereas others do not. They include proprioceptive neuromuscular facilitation (PNF), myofascial release, dynamic stretching, ballistic stretching, and active isolated stretching. This book focuses on static stretching because it's ideal for at-home solo workouts that focus on pain relief and prevention.

Techniques

If you are just starting out with this program, you'll want to work your way up to a 30-second hold. Start with 10 to 15 seconds and add 5 seconds every session until you get to 30. A longer hold is more effective.

Seven muscles are very important as movers and stabilizers of the lower back and pelvis: gluteals, tensor fasciae latae, hamstrings, quadriceps, adductors, psoas, and piriformis. To ensure you have the recipe for success, I've put together a stretch for each of them.

PIGEON GLUTE STRETCH

EASY

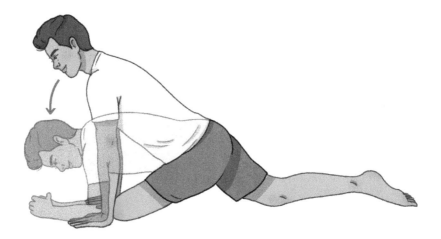

When you sit for most of the day, your gluteals (buttocks) can become tight and weak. The gluteals are attached to the pelvis, and over time, the tightness and weakness can cause lower back pain and dysfunction.

As you compensate for gluteal problems, you can set off a chain reaction where you may naturally rotate your pelvis, which leads to one hip elevating and the leg on that side essentially becoming shorter as a result. That can affect your walking and running, which creates additional problems for your pelvis and causes additional back pain.

This stretch works the glutes and opens up the joint spaces of the lumbar spine, which can greatly relieve lower back tension. It's a favorite among many of my patients. If you do yoga, you may recognize this stretch as a modification of pigeon pose.

Instructions:

1. Position yourself on all fours.

2. Bring your left knee forward and rest it on the floor.

3. Cross your left knee over your right leg.

4. Let your right knee touch the ground.

5. Drop your torso forward, toward the floor. The more you drop your torso, the deeper a stretch you'll get on your left glute.

6. Breathe and relax. Let gravity do the work as you hold for 20 to 30 seconds.

7. Alternate sides.

8. Repeat three times on each side.

STAY SAFE:

Your body will stop you from folding up like a pretzel if you're not flexible enough to do so. Don't force it. You don't want to injure yourself by trying to bend your leg in a way it hasn't bent in years (or decades).

EASY DOES IT:

At first, you may not be flexible enough to fold your front leg as instructed. That's okay. Work your way to that point, getting your leg as close to the ideal position as you can. You also may not be able to drop your torso too far forward at first. Go as far as you can and aim to drop even lower next time.

TFL WALL STRETCH

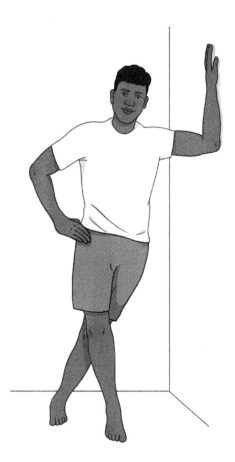

The tensor fasciae latae (TFL) is one of your upper thigh muscles. It acts on your iliotibial (IT) band, which is the connective tissue sheath (fascia) that runs down the side of your thigh, past your knee, and serves quite a few functions for your pelvis, hips, and legs.

    Like the glutes, the TFL tightens when you sit too much. And as with other muscles attached to the pelvis, that tightness can cause problems with the joints above and below the muscle itself. That's how a tight TFL in your leg can cause pain in your back.

Instructions:

1. Stand next to a wall, sideways, slightly less than an arm's length away. Begin with your right side facing the wall.

2. Reach out your right arm to balance against the wall.

3. Cross your left leg across your right leg.

4. Keep your lower back in arched (extended) position.

5. Let your pelvis lean toward the wall, as if you'd bump the wall with your hip if you got closer.

6. You will begin to feel the stretch as you lean in. When you do, hold for 20 to 30 seconds.

7. Repeat three times on each side.

STAY SAFE:

Make sure you're balanced. You don't want to fall or crash into the wall because you leaned too far.

EASY DOES IT:

The farther you lean your pelvis, the more of a stretch you'll feel. While a deeper lean will be more effective, if you need to begin with less of a lean as you build up your flexibility, stamina, balance, and workout confidence, you can modify your position accordingly.

TFL FOAM ROLLING

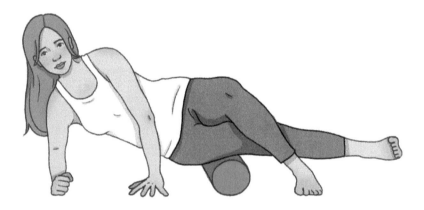

Here's another way to loosen the TFL, which is a notoriously difficult muscle to relax, as well as the glutes. A foam roller is a low-cost, low-tech self-help solution that can help you relieve your lower back pain symptoms. This maneuver is more advanced, however, so attempt it only after you've graduated up to the medium or advanced program.

I recommend a foam roller with a six-inch diameter. You can get one at any exercise equipment store or purchase one online.

Instructions:

1. Lie on your right side and prop yourself up with your elbow.

2. Place the roller perpendicular to your body, over the center of the TFL. You will also be making contact with the gluteals.

3. Relax your shoulder and allow your body to drop onto the roller.

4. You will feel increasing pressure as you drop, and it may become slightly painful. At the pain point, push up ever so slightly, breathe into the pressure, and hold the position for 5 to 10 seconds.

5. Slowly roll and lean back so you can work on the rest of the muscle. In two to three minutes, you should be able to cover the entire muscle.

6. Switch to your left side and repeat.

STAY SAFE:

In the gym I often see people use the roller to work on the IT band itself. I don't recommend doing so because the tissue is very thin, and pressure can cause an irritation that outweighs the benefits of rolling. I recommend using a foam roller on the muscle itself, as opposed to connective tissue.

EASY DOES IT:

This stretch requires a lot of balance and some slight pain. You can mitigate balance or pain issues by resting the top part of your body on your mat. Doing so takes the pressure off your TFL, so it decreases the effectiveness of the foam rolling. Use this technique to get situated and comfortable with the foam rolling motion, then try to elevate yourself properly.

PSOAS DOORWAY STRETCH

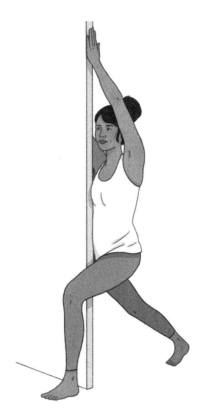

When patients complain of lower back pain, I always check their psoas muscle, as tightness is often a culprit. The psoas muscle goes from your spine through your pelvis to your femur and is the primary connection between your torso and your legs. It's responsible for quite a bit of your bending and leg movement.

The psoas can get tight from both sedentary work and heavy manual labor. When you sit all day, your hips are in the flexed position, which gradually tightens the muscle. In the same way, bending over all day to use, say, a jackhammer can cause the same problem. It's often hard for people to accept that working at a computer can be as dangerous to the lower back as working a jackhammer, but it's true.

Instructions:

1. Stand in a doorway so the right side of your body is pressed against the doorjamb and your left leg is extended through the doorway.

2. Bring your right leg back two to three feet.

3. Stand on your toes, with your heels off the floor.

4. Bring your arms above your head and place them on the wall above you.

5. Bend your knees slightly.

6. As you begin to feel the stretching of the psoas on the right side of your abdomen, hold the position for 20 to 30 seconds.

7. Repeat three times on each side.

STAY SAFE:

Make sure you feel balanced before you begin to stretch. Don't skip putting your arms on the wall. This step ensures you don't topple over.

EASY DOES IT:

The less you extend your right leg backward, the easier this stretch will be. You want to work your way up to the recommended two to three feet, but if this distance is too taxing to begin with, a shorter distance will work. You can also try this stretch flat-footed, rather than on your toes, as you learn the proper positioning and motion.

HAMSTRING DOORWAY STRETCH

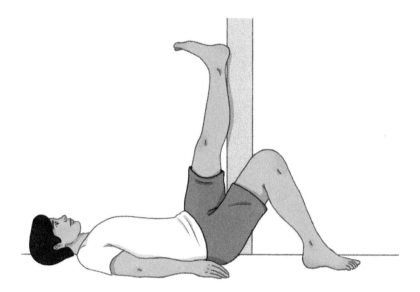

Your hamstring muscles are on the back of your thigh and perform two important functions: They extend the hip and flex the knee. If your hamstrings are tighter than normal, your pelvis may be forced backward, which causes a whole host of problems.

I see it happen all the time: Patients come to me with lower back pain, I prescribe leg stretches, and they say, "Doc, I don't understand. Why are you giving me leg stretches when my lower back hurts?" I explain that, because many of the muscles of the legs connect to the pelvis and the lumbar spine sits on that pelvis, the flexibility and strength of those leg muscles will directly impact the lower back.

When I examine my patients, hamstring tightness is one of my most common findings. Most of the patients I see in my San Francisco office are tech workers who sit all day with their knees flexed, which causes their hamstrings to shorten.

This hamstring stretch is a one-person version of a common two-person hamstring stretch where one person lies on their back with a leg in the air, and the other person stands above them, pushing on that leg.

There are multiple ways to stretch the hamstrings, but I opt for this one because it requires the least physical effort, which allows you to relax into the stretch.

Instructions:

1. Lie on your back in a doorway with your left leg up on the doorjamb.

2. Extend your right leg through the doorway.

3. Bend your right leg at the knee to stabilize your lower back and keep it flat on the ground.

4. Position your buttocks as close as you can to the doorjamb. The closer you are, the deeper the stretch.

5. Continue to a point where you feel the restriction, then push a bit more. Remember, don't stretch into pain.

6. Hold for 30 seconds.

7. Repeat three times on each leg.

STAY SAFE:

You want to push a very small amount past the point where you feel restriction from your hamstring. "Very small" is an important designation. You can risk injury if you let the wall push your hamstring too far.

EASY DOES IT:

While you want to position your buttocks as close to the door as possible, you may find it easier at first to be a little farther away. Your leg may not be ready for a 90-degree angle on day one of an exercise program.

STANDING QUADRICEPS STRETCH

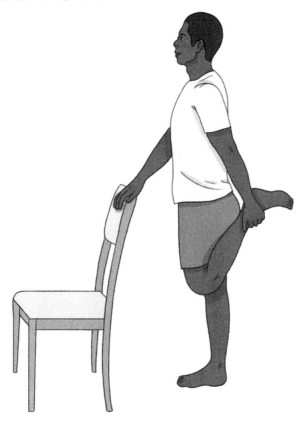

The quadriceps muscle, on the front of your thigh, is made of four components (thus the "quad" designation). It allows you to bend your hip and straighten your knee. It's a very important muscle for basic daily activities like getting up from a chair or going up and down stairs.

Just like tight hamstrings can pull the pelvis backward, tight quadriceps can pull the pelvis forward. Hypertonic (overly tight) quadriceps can cause pain and dysfunction of the knee, the hip, and the pelvis, as well as any other joints above or below the muscle.

Instructions:

1. Bend your left leg backward and grab your left ankle.

2. Pull your leg toward your buttocks until you feel a tightening of the muscle.

3. Once you feel the tension, continue to pull back just a touch more.

4. Hold for 20 to 30 seconds.

5. Repeat three times on each leg.

STAY SAFE:

Much like the hamstring stretch, when you pull back your leg, go only a small amount past the point at which you feel tension. If you pull too hard, you could risk injury.

EASY DOES IT:

It can be challenging to maintain your balance while doing this stretch. If you're having trouble, try holding onto a chair or doorjamb for stability.

BUTTERFLY ADDUCTORS STRETCH

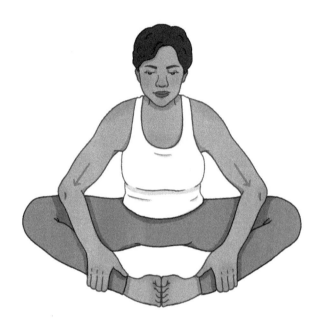

Your legs can move in six different directions: forward (flexion), backward (extension), left rotation, right rotation, away from the center of your body (abduction), and toward the center of your body (adduction). The group of muscles called the adductors are responsible for pulling the thigh toward the center of the body at the hip joint.

Weak or tight adductors can lead to stability issues with your hips, which in turn can cause lower back pain.

Instructions:

1. Begin by sitting on the floor.

2. Bend both knees so the soles of your feet are touching in front of you, ankles against the floor.

3. Hold your ankles with both hands.

4. Place your elbows where they naturally land on your knees.

5. Bend forward slowly from your waist, simultaneously pushing down on your knees with the elbows, and hold for 20 to 30 seconds.

6. Repeat three times.

STAY SAFE:

This is a very safe stretch that is hard to overdo, but make sure you're not pushing your knees down too much with your elbows to the point where you feel pain.

EASY DOES IT:

Ideally, you'd fold yourself all the way forward in this stretch. If that's not realistic, bend forward as far as you can.

LYING LEG REST PIRIFORMIS STRETCH

EASY

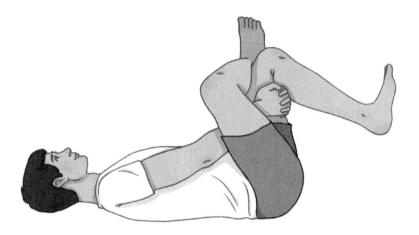

The piriformis is a muscle in the gluteal region that's responsible for lateral thigh rotation and abduction. The sciatic nerve passes underneath it, so when the muscle is tight or in spasm, it can put pressure on the nerve and cause a great deal of buttock and leg pain.

Because the piriformis is underneath the glutes, the stretch to loosen it is similar to the glute stretch.

Instructions:

1. Lie on your back with both knees bent and your feet flat on the floor.

2. Bring up your left leg and place your left ankle on your right knee.

3. Take hold of your right thigh.

4. Pull your right knee gently toward your chest.

5. As you feel the stretch, pull just a touch further. Hold this position for 20 to 30 seconds.

6. Repeat two or three times on each side.

STAY SAFE:

When the piriformis becomes hyper-tonic or goes into a spasm, you can develop piriformis syndrome, which is pain in the buttocks that radiates down the leg. Poor exercise form can cause this condition, so always be mindful of how you might be subtly hurting yourself. For example, when running, avoid uneven surfaces and stretch before and after. As for safety during the stretch itself, as always, go only a slight bit past your point of resistance. Don't pull too far and risk an injury.

EASY DOES IT:

This stretch involves folding yourself up into something of a knot. If you don't have the flexibility to do so at first, bring your leg up as best you can and fold it as much as possible.

CHAPTER 6

Strengthening

CAT/COW 78

KNEE-TO-CHEST STRETCH AND PELVIC TILTS 80

CURL-UP 82

PRESS-UP, OR MODIFIED COBRA 84

THE CRUNCH 86

SUPINE TWIST 88

FACEDOWN (PRONE) BACK EXTENSION 90

FACEUP (SUPINE) BACK EXTENSION 92

ALTERNATING LEG BALANCE 94

THE CROSS CRAWL 96

DEAD BUG 98

BASIC PLANK 102

SIDE PLANK 104

CRUNCH WITH EXERCISE BALL 106

SUPINE TWIST WITH EXERCISE BALL 108

FACEDOWN (PRONE) BACK EXTENSION WITH EXERCISE BALL 110

FACEUP (SUPINE) BACK EXTENSION WITH EXERCISE BALL 112

ALTERNATING LEG BALANCE WITH BALANCE PAD 114

CROSS CRAWL WITH EXERCISE BALL 116

DEAD BUG WITH FOAM ROLLER 118

CLIMBING PLANK 122

PLANK WITH LEG EXTENSIONS 124

STAGGERED PLANK 126

CROSS CLIMBER 128

JACKKNIFE WITH PUSH-UP 130

EXERCISE BALL PUSH-UP 132

ALTERNATING LEG BALANCE WITH ROCKER BOARD OR FOAM ROLLER 134

HANGING LEG RAISE 136

BANANA ROLL 138

The single most important way to heal and prevent back pain is to develop a strong and balanced core. The core is a set of 29 muscles that controls the lumbo-pelvic-hip complex. It's your center of gravity and the place where much of your movement originates. The core is an integrated, functional unit made up of your abdominal muscles on the front and sides of your torso, the paraspinal erector muscles that keep you upright, and the many other muscles that connect to your lumbar spines, pelvic bones, and femurs. Your core also includes the diaphragm, which is your breathing muscle, as well as long attachments of muscles like the tensor fasciae latae and hamstrings that go below your knees to your leg bones (tibia). Strengthening this area involves much more than developing a six-pack.

You move many core muscles unconsciously and involuntarily, so you probably think about them rarely, if ever. But they are extremely important in stabilizing the joints of your spine and allowing forces to move and transfer through those joints.

In this context, "stabilizing" refers to your coordination and balance. Your muscles work together in a highly sophisticated manner. To perform certain actions, when one muscle is activated, another might need to slow down. Muscles work together (synergistically) or in opposition to one another (antagonistically). When the dance isn't coordinated properly, the forces don't move smoothly through your joints, which makes you more susceptible to injury and pain.

The core provides important protection for the spine during everyday activities that can injure you, like bending, sitting, lifting, and running. A core stabilization and strengthening program helps you gain strength, control, and endurance.

In many ways, your core acts like the foundation of your home. It not only protects your lower back but also helps support everything that sits above it. For example, perhaps one day you notice that one of the shingles on the roof of your house came loose and fell to the ground, so you go up to the roof and replace it. A month later, it happens again, except this time two shingles come down. When you tell a building contractor what's been going on, he asks you to show him your basement. You're skeptical—after all, you have a roof problem and the basement is at the absolute opposite end of the house—but you let him take a look. When he inspects your foundation, he sees a big crack that has allowed your home to shift. This crack is your roof problem.

You can experience the same phenomenon in your body. Pay attention after you do a set of abdominal exercises (and you will have plenty to choose from in this section), and you'll find you're naturally standing more upright. It's because of a muscular connection between the core muscles and the mid- and upper-back muscles, as well as a neurological connection that helps coordinate all their movements.

I always remind my patients that "the back has a front." The coordinated work from front to back and inside to outside helps keep you safe and pain-free. In this chapter, we'll be going through a series of exercises you can mix and match, with a focus on strengthening your core by working your lumbar and abdominal muscles.

Tools

I am a big advocate of low-cost, low-tech self-help tools. Even with a minimal amount of space in your home, you can put together a mini gym that will work for the exercises, stretches, and strengthening techniques described throughout this book.

You can also add some tools to your mini gym to help your exercise and recovery process even more. Some of the tools and equipment that I recommend include:

Exercise ball. For strengthening and stabilizing the lower back, the most valuable tool is the simple exercise ball (also known as a physioball). You can use this inflatable ball to perform a variety of exercises, many of which are described in this book.

Many of the strengthening exercises in the medium and hard workout programs incorporate the exercise ball. If you invest in only one tool on this list, make it this one. It's inexpensive and readily available online and in sporting goods stores. Your height and the exercises you'll be doing will determine the size of ball you need.

A word of caution: Exercise balls can take a bit of work to inflate. They come with a hand or foot pump, but I recommend going to a local gas station, paying the 50 cents at the air station, putting the compressor nozzle over the receptacle on the ball, and letting it do the work. The ball will be full within 30 seconds. This option will be especially helpful if you are having any pain in your lower back or shoulder. After all, there's nothing more frustrating than injuring your back when you're blowing up a device you bought to heal your back.

Exercises for Seniors

Physical activity is important for people of all ages. It is especially important as you grow older and want to keep doing the things you love to do, whether playing tennis, gardening, going to a playground with the grandkids, or simply taking walks in the park. Unfortunately, lower back pain can get in the way of enjoying the activities that make life meaningful.

The needs of seniors can be unique because of a lifetime of wear and tear on the body. Joints and muscles naturally stiffen with age, and the cardiovascular system becomes sluggish. It is important to move to counteract this natural process.

Before you start an exercise program, consult with your physician. Make sure you don't have any health issues that would limit you or prohibit you from doing any particular activities.

Once you get the all-clear from your doctor, ease into your exercise plan. Your areas of focus should be strength, endurance, flexibility, and balance.

To improve strength, do resistance training with weights, bands, or your own body weight. Endurance comes from cardio exercise. Flexibility is the result of a commitment to stretching. And balance is the result of channeling your strength, endurance, and flexibility into balance-building exercises.

While you're almost certainly reading this book because of past or present lower back pain, the benefits of this whole-body approach can extend even further. Strength, endurance, flexibility, and balance can decrease your risk of developing chronic diseases, like diabetes and high blood pressure. They can increase your ability to perform necessary tasks like walking up stairs and carrying groceries and minimize your chance of falls. And they improve your quality of life because you can move through your day-to-day activities pain-free.

Plus, you can have fun while you're doing it! Find activities you enjoy, like swimming, biking, or even playing basketball. Carry your grandchildren. Practice yoga. Take up tai chi.

When I walk through the parks of Chinatown in San Francisco, I often see groups of seniors practicing tai chi. It almost looks like a beautiful slow-motion dance. Tai chi is a whole-body exercise that combines balance, flexibility, and strength. And because it is done so slowly, there is no danger of injuring joints with high impact. It's also very relaxing and is often referred to as a moving meditation.

Your body was meant to move. When you stop, things break down—sometimes quickly. But you can build it up again. It's never too late.

Feel free to start with the easy strength program in this book. Choose a cardio activity you enjoy. Build strength by walking up and down stairs or start using small handheld weights. Try yoga stretches to loosen up your muscles and mobilize your joints. And do some crunches so you can get that six-pack you always wanted (just kidding!). I promise after the core workout you will stand taller and feel a bit more energy. And yes, you may even get some relief from that low-grade nagging back pain.

You will feel better when you move. And there is no better time to start than right now.

Foam roller. No home workout space is complete without a foam roller. I generally recommend one with a six-inch diameter and 36-inch length. The roller can serve multiple functions. It's great for stretching and self-massaging muscles; I especially like it for getting into the gluteals and the tensor fasciae latae. It is also great for adding another level of challenge when you're doing exercises that require balance. Because it is a cylinder, when you lie on your back with the roller between your body and the floor, it will make any exercise more challenging.

A handful of exercises in the medium and hard workout programs incorporate the foam roller. But you can still get a lot of use out of a foam roller when you're doing the easy program, thanks to its stretching and massage applications.

Balance pad. You will also be focusing on lower back stability, so it's important to work on balance. The body works as a kinetic chain, meaning the various body parts have interrelationships with one another. An unstable foot or ankle, whether the result of old or new injuries, can impact the joints above the area of injury, from the knee to the hip to the sacroiliac and lumbar spine. A balance pad is a simple foam pad of varying densities that can assist in strengthening and stabilizing the foot and ankle to support the lower back. One exercise in the medium section incorporates the balance pad.

Pull-up bar. There are plenty of places you can find pull-up bars, like gyms or even local playgrounds. But if you want to set up a mini gym in your home, look into installing your own. Many can be mounted securely in a door frame and will save you a trip outside your house.

You may be thinking, "Pull-up bar? I'm not doing pull-ups! Also, how will those help my lower back?" This question will be answered in the hard workout program. One of the exercises incorporates the pull-up bar.

Self-massagers. Self-massage tools like a Theracane (a plastic hook-shaped device) or the more expensive Theragun can be used to target tight, painful areas of muscular tension. Many people swear by the latter, so if you have the budget and you want the most powerful at-home massage tool available, the investment may be worthwhile. But the Theracane also gets the job done.

Bands. An elastic resistance band is another helpful tool for improving strength and balance. These bands vary in tension, so you can graduate from light resistance to strong. If you enjoy working with resistance and have the space, you can step up to a TRX system, which provides increased variation because of the heavy-duty resistance of the TRX bands. You will be able to hang in different planes of movement, thus adding your body weight into the mix. While none of the workouts in this book explicitly includes bands or the TRX system, as you vary your workouts in the future or need to increase the challenge on your stretches, bands are an inexpensive but effective solution.

Weights. Another simple, low-cost enhancement to your workout is the basic free weight. Dumbbells start at one pound and are often sold by the pound. By adding handheld free weights to some of the exercises in this book, you can increase both repetitions and resistance. Over time, you can graduate to kettlebells, which are handheld bell-shaped weights that can help you develop additional core power.

Medicine balls. You can also consider adding one or more weighted medicine balls to your workouts. They come in a variety of weights, usually starting at two pounds and going up to 12 pounds. Medicine balls provide a significant advantage over dumbbells and kettlebells: You can throw them around without putting a hole through your wall. One exercise, which strengthens the transverse abdominal muscles, involves standing sideways about six feet from a wall. Holding the medicine ball and throwing it against the wall as you rotate your trunk is a great way to strengthen the side muscles. But don't try it with a kettlebell!

Inflatable cushion. You can even strengthen and balance your core while you're sitting at your desk. A simple inflatable cushion can be used on the seat of your chair. It moves very slightly beneath you and helps firm up the core as you work.

Please note: You absolutely don't have to rush out and spend hundreds or thousands of dollars on equipment. You can complete a program of healthy back strengthening using just your body weight and the floor. But as you continue to progress in your stretching and strength training and you want to up your challenge, diversify your routine, and improve your results, you can gradually add in more tools or equipment as you see fit.

Techniques

I've put together three strengthening programs: easy, medium, and hard. I recommend trying and mastering the easy ones before moving on to medium and hard.

Ideally, you should do this strengthening program three or four times per week, mixed in with the stretching and cardio exercise in the previous chapter to promote a whole-body musculoskeletal approach to healthy back care.

Also, note that some of the exercises, especially in the easy program, fall in a middle ground between stretching and strengthening. For the purposes of the book, I am including a few in the strengthening section as they're just a bit more oriented toward strength than flexibility.

CAT/COW

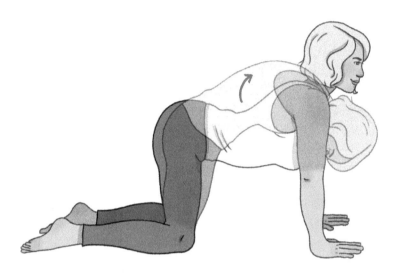

The cat/cow falls somewhere between a stretch and a strengthening exercise. It is a very gentle movement that helps loosen up the joints of the lumbar spine, improve posture, and support balance. This movement will be incorporated into other, more challenging exercises.

Instructions:

1. Position yourself on all fours.

2. Relax and let your lower back/lumbar spine drop toward the floor. (This is cow position.)

3. Tighten your abdominal muscles and round your lower back. (This is cat position.)

4. Focus on your breathing throughout the movements.

5. Repeat 5 to 10 times.

STAY SAFE:

This is a gentle, simple exercise, but if you feel any pain, stop immediately.

EASY DOES IT:

As you drop and raise your lower back, you may find your movements are slight. Build up to a deeper drop and more rounded arch.

KNEE-TO-CHEST STRETCH AND PELVIC TILTS

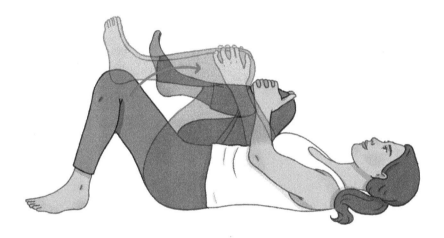

Knee-to-chest stretches and pelvic tilts can be very helpful for relieving lower back pain, but they aren't appropriate for everyone. If your practitioner has determined that a bulging disc is causing your pain, these stretches can actually increase that bulge. (Picture a water balloon: When you press on the front, it bulges backward. The same thing happens with these stretches and a bulging disc.)

But if your pain is coming from the back of the lumbar joint segment, around the facets, these stretches can take pressure off those irritated nerves, relieving your pain.

Instructions:

Knee-to-chest stretch:

1. Lie on your back with both knees bent.

2. Bring your left knee up toward your chest.

3. Hold your left knee.

4. While you continue to hold your left knee, bring the right knee up.

Pelvic tilt:

1. Stay in the same position.

2. Keep your knees bent and gently press your lower back against the floor. (It won't have a long way to go!)

3. Hold for two or three seconds, then release.

4. Repeat 5 to 10 times.

5. Hold both knees and pull them down toward your chest.

6. Hold for a few seconds.

7. Bring one knee down to the floor, followed by the other.

8. Repeat 5 to 10 times.

STAY SAFE:

It is very common for people to receive a sheet of lower back exercises from their health-care practitioner when they come to the office with lower back pain. But stretches and exercises aren't a one-size-fits-all prescription. It is important to determine which movements are appropriate for *you*. If you have a bulging disc, some stretches can make it worse.

EASY DOES IT:

You may not be able to get your knees all the way to your chest. Just pull them as far as you can.

CURL-UP

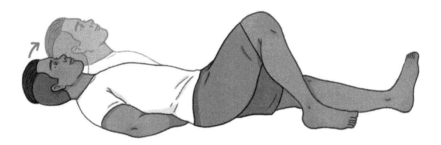

This is a very gentle, subtle exercise that teaches you to engage your core with a physical challenge. In my practice, I see many people who are disconnected from their body. They aren't literally disconnected, of course, but they lack the ability to move their body in a conscious way. They experience a kind of incoordination in which the body does not seem able to follow the commands of the mind. It becomes most apparent when I am instructing them on how to make subtle movements that are not physically difficult.

The curl-up is one example of a subtle movement. It seems simple, but it takes real perseverance for many people to get it right.

Instructions:

1. Lie on your back with your knees bent and feet flat on the floor.

2. Place your hands under your lower back, finding the curve of your lumbar spine.

3. Straighten one leg while keeping the other knee bent. Your hands should feel the lower back muscles tightening. As they do, make sure the curve of your lower back does not change.

4. Breathe in.

5. As you exhale, gently lift your head off the floor without altering the curve of your lower back.

6. Hold the position for six to eight seconds.

7. Bring your head back to the floor and your knee back to a bent position.

8. Repeat 5 to 10 times, with each leg extended.

PRESS-UP, OR MODIFIED COBRA

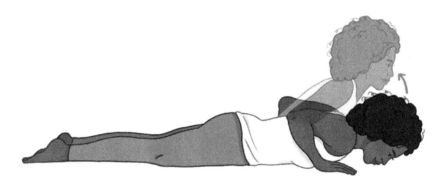

If your pain is the result of an irritated disc, you will most likely benefit from this movement. Going back to the water balloon analogy, pressing on the back of the balloon will cause it to bulge forward. If posterior disc irritation is causing pain, this stretch will provide relief by taking pressure off the nerve root.

You may recognize this as a modification of the classic yoga pose called cobra. In the classic cobra, you hold your position at the end point of the stretch. In this version, the movement should be continuous. The intention is to pump the disc.

Instructions:

1. Lie facedown on the floor.

2. Relax your lower back. Taking a few breaths can help with relaxation.

3. Gently press your torso up with your arms, being mindful that all the work with this stretch should come from the arms, passively arching your lower back.

4. Gently reverse and lower down.

5. Repeat 5 to 10 times.

STAY SAFE:

Don't tense your lower back. You want your arms to do the work, and if your lower back gets involved, you're not stretching it properly.

EASY DOES IT:

Bend as much as you can comfortably while maintaining proper form.

THE CRUNCH

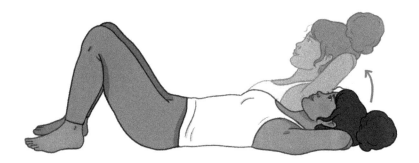

One of the clinics I work in specializes in treating work-related injuries. There, I see the heavy lifters: the steel workers wielding blowtorches all day; the drivers of the beer delivery trucks who haul kegs from the distributor's loading dock to the truck to the local bar; the housekeepers in the hotels, turning mattresses and changing sheets in dozens of rooms; the cops; the firefighters; the tree trimmers.

When they come to see me, I ask if they are exercising. They generally look at me like I'm crazy. Some say, "Doc, are you nuts? Do I exercise? I lift kegs of beer all day. So, yes, I exercise." Or, "I flip mattresses all day. Of course I'm exercising." And although it is certainly true that they are doing exercise by lifting heavy weights, walking, and so on, almost none of them is doing the exercise they need to do: core strengthening and stabilization. Strengthening your abdominals is an essential part of a back pain prevention program. Crunches allow you to work on these muscles safely.

There are several groups of abdominal muscles: transverse, rectus, and obliques. Even though they're at the front of your body, they work hand in hand with the lower back muscles. Think of the muscles as being part of your internal lumbar supports (which is why I discourage the use of lumbar belts unless you're in acute pain).

Instructions:

1. Lie on your back with your knees bent and feet flat on the floor.

2. Lift your torso approximately 25 to 30 degrees, which is less than halfway to vertical. Go just until you feel a tightening sensation in your belly. Once you do, lift only a few more degrees.

3. Repeat 5 to 10 times.

Once you have done this exercise comfortably for a few days, add a slight variation. On your first repetition, come straight up as described. With the second rep, come up and gently rotate your torso, twisting so your right elbow points to your left knee. On the next rep, do the opposite, with your left elbow pointing to your right knee. With this addition, you will be engaging both the rectus abdominus muscles and the obliques.

STAY SAFE:

Remember, the exercise is meant to strengthen the abdominal muscles, not the back muscles. When you are doing the crunches, you should mainly feel a tightening in the front of your torso, not in your back. If you feel an uncomfortable tension in your lower back, ease back a few degrees until it releases. Do not lift your body past this point.

If you have neck pain, you can do a reverse crunch. Start in the same position, lying on your back with your knees bent and feet flat on the floor, but instead of bringing your torso toward your knees, bring your knees toward your torso. Slowly bring both knees up to your chest and then back to the floor. This modification allows you to contract the abdominals without putting any strain on your neck and upper back.

EASY DOES IT:

Take your time. There is no reason to rush. When you stand up, you will feel like you are standing more upright. (And you are!)

SUPINE TWIST

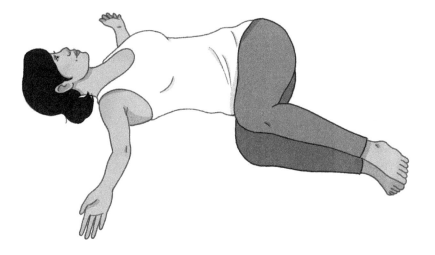

This exercise is another easy way to work your transverse and oblique abdominals. You are building up your internal support by strengthening all the muscles that wrap around your abdomen.

Instructions:

1. Lie on your back with your knees bent and feet flat on the floor.

2. Slowly, with your knees together and mindfully engaging your abdominal muscles, lower your knees to the left, until you have gone as close as you can to the floor.

3. Hold in that position for three or four seconds.

4. Slowly bring the knees back past starting position and lower them to the right, until you have gone as close as you can to the floor.

5. Repeat 10 to 15 times.

STAY SAFE:

As with the previous exercise, you should feel tightening in your abdominal muscles, not your back. If you feel it in your back, you're probably pushing too far and not maintaining proper form.

EASY DOES IT:

You don't have to touch your knees to the floor to benefit from this exercise. Just lower your knees as far as you can. If you feel the stretch in your abdomen (and if you are a little sore in your side abs the next day), the stretch is working.

FACEDOWN (PRONE) BACK EXTENSION

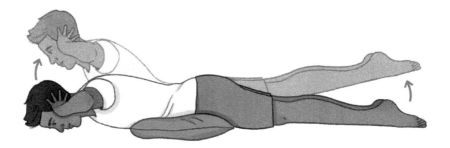

Your torso muscles are your lumbar supports. With a strong internal lumbar support, you can move more freely and safely through your normal ranges of motion because your muscles are on the front lines protecting you.

Picture a tube of toothpaste. When you put your hand around the middle of the tube and squeeze, the paste above your hand is pushed up and the paste below your hand moves down. The same thing happens when you tighten your core. You are effectively elongating your spine and relieving the pressure on your intervertebral joints. This motion may relieve pain and help prevent the ongoing irritation of those joints. You're slowing down the wear and tear that contributes to dysfunction and pain.

But it's not enough to work only on your abs, no matter what the '80s exercise equipment infomercials told you. You also need to strengthen the lower back itself. This back extension exercise is the first step.

Instructions:

1. Lie facedown on the floor with a pillow under your abdomen.

2. Place your hands at your side or grasp them behind your neck.

3. Gently lift your torso off the floor.

4. Hold for three to five seconds.

5. Relax, returning your torso to the floor.

6. Repeat 5 to 10 times.

Once you feel comfortable and strong after a few days of doing this exercise, add one more movement into the mix. As you lift your torso off the floor, lift both legs as well so your back forms a nice curve. You'll look like a bowl, with your upper back and legs forming the edges of that bowl.

A good modification of this exercise is to lift one leg at a time, rather than both simultaneously. This movement will improve your balance as well as your strength. You can also try the exercise with your arms at your side and then extended straight above your head.

STAY SAFE:

These exercises should never cause sharp pain. If you feel that kind of pain, stop right away. But keep in mind when you're using muscles that have been dormant for a while, it's not unusual to feel some light soreness during and after the exercise. As you get stronger, the discomfort should pass in a day or two. If it doesn't, stop doing the exercise and consult your health-care practitioner.

EASY DOES IT:

The goal of this exercise, and many others, is not to go as far as you can into any particular movement, but rather to contract the targeted muscles in a sustained, healthy manner. There are no prizes for pushing yourself to the absolute end of your range of motion, but there are great rewards for building up your strength gradually by steadily increasing your repetitions.

FACEUP (SUPINE) BACK EXTENSION

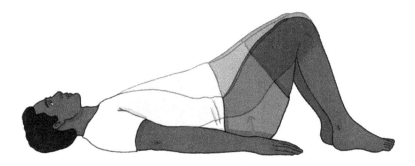

Now that you've strengthened your back while lying facedown, it's time to reverse. Lying faceup will activate and challenge your muscles in a different way, and this variation is key to building strength.

Instructions:

1. Lie on your back on the floor with your knees slightly bent.

2. Lift your pelvis off the floor as high as you can. Your upper back should remain flat on the floor.

3. Hold for three to five seconds.

4. Bring your pelvis back down to the floor.

5. Repeat 10 to 15 times.

STAY SAFE:

This is a very safe exercise, so you don't have to worry too much when you're performing it. But, as always, if anything feels off as you're lifting your pelvis, stop doing the exercise.

EASY DOES IT:

As much as you'll want to lift your pelvis as high in the air as you can, take it slow. Remember, your upper back needs to stay on the floor. If it starts to elevate, you're lifting too high.

ALTERNATING LEG BALANCE

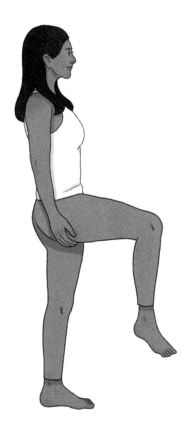

One common cause of lower back pain can be traced to the feet and ankles, so I always include them when I examine a patient with lower back pain.

    This simple test can tell you whether if you have an underlying foot or ankle issue you need to address. In the standing position, with eyes open, lift your leg, bent at the knee, and hold for as long as you can, up to 30 seconds. Repeat the same action with the other leg. Repeat the movements, this time with your eyes closed.

Once you take your eyes out of the equation, it is almost always more difficult to maintain your balance. The extent of the difference between your balance with your eyes open and closed will give you an idea of how much rehabilitative work you need to do on your feet and ankles.

Have you ever sprained your ankle? In the process, you damaged some nerve endings called proprioceptors. This damage caused a disruption of the signaling pathway from the end of your extremity to the brain and back down. As a result, the little muscles lost their ability to fire off in a coordinated manner, making it much more likely you'll roll your ankle again.

The following exercises can help rehabilitate your foot and ankle and regenerate the damaged proprioceptors.

Instructions:

1. In a standing position, lift one leg, bent at the knee. Your thigh should be perpendicular to the floor, with your calf at a 90-degree angle to it.

2. Hold the position for up to 30 seconds.

3. Repeat with the opposite leg.

4. Once you are able to hold the position for 30 seconds on each leg, repeat the exercise with your eyes closed until you are able to maintain balance for 30 seconds.

STAY SAFE:

This exercise can be really tricky (doing things with your eyes closed usually is). Take care not to fall down. Be sure to stand next to a fixed surface or object so if you do stumble, you have something to grab.

EASY DOES IT:

The purpose behind this exercise is to improve balance, strengthen the feet and ankles, and help heal and prevent the onset of lower back pain. If you have knee or hip pain, it may not be possible to bend your knee and hip to a 90-degree angle. That's fine. The main goal is balance. Even if you lift your leg off the ground just a few inches, you will still be getting the benefit of balancing, stabilizing, and strengthening the ankles and feet.

THE CROSS CRAWL

EASY

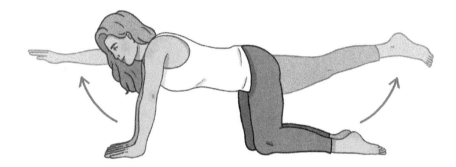

It's important to reiterate that a solid core requires strength and balance, and this exercise improves both.

One of the great things about this exercise is, like the previous one, you'll get immediate feedback. You'll see how unbalanced you are, but also how quickly you can improve.

The exercise uses two positions: cat and cow. For cat, you'll be on your hands and knees with your lower back rounded toward the ceiling. For cow, you'll relax your lower back and let your lumbar spine drop toward the floor. Before you dive into this exercise, get comfortable moving from the cat position to the cow position (see page 78).

Instructions:

1. Start in the cat position (on your hands and knees, lower back rounded toward the ceiling).

2. Lift your right arm in front of you.

3. Hold your arm straight out for three to five seconds.

4. Bring your hand back to the floor.

5. Do the same movement with the left arm, again holding for three to five seconds before bringing your hand back to the floor.

6. Bring the right leg straight out behind you.

7. Hold for three to five seconds.

8. Bring your knee back to the floor.

9. Do the same movement with the left leg, again holding for three to five seconds before bringing your knee back to the floor.

10. Lift the left arm and the right leg at the same time and hold for three to five seconds before returning them to the floor.

11. Lift the right arm and the left leg at the same time and hold for three to five seconds before returning them to the floor.

12. Repeat the sequence three times.

13. Do the entire sequence again, this time in the cow position.

14. Repeat the sequence three times.

STAY SAFE:

Some people have a hard time with this exercise. You may not be able to hold your arms or legs in position without feeling like you will fall over. The reaction is to retreat back to the stable position on all fours, especially when lifting the opposite arm and leg. This exercise vividly illustrates any lack of coordination of the muscles that keep your core balanced and functioning as an integrated unit. To master the exercise (that is, avoid tipping over), you must engage the core muscles. You will feel your abdominal and paraspinal muscles tighten up automatically. If they don't, you will lose your balance.

EASY DOES IT:

It's okay if you can hold your arm or leg up for only one or two seconds at first or if you can't hold them up at all. If you persist, your balance will improve quickly. Then you'll be ready to make the exercise even more challenging, as we'll cover in the medium difficulty workout program.

DEAD BUG

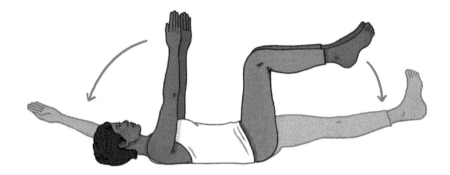

This exercise is also great for your core and involves both physical strength and coordination. It focuses on the deep core muscles: the transverse abdominis and the erectors. It also combines strengthening with coordination by engaging contralateral (opposite leg and arm) movement at the same time.

Instructions:

1. Lie on your back on the floor, with your arms straight up over your chest. Your arms should be at a 90-degree angle with your torso.

2. Bring your hips toward your chest so your thighs make a right angle with your pelvis. At the same time, your knees should also be bent at right angles. (You should look like, well, a dead bug.)

3. Press your lower back flat against the floor to engage your core. Throughout this exercise, be mindful of maintaining this position.

4. Slowly bring your right arm down so it's nearly touching the floor. Your arm should be parallel with your body with your palm facing up.

5. At the same time, bring your left leg down, extending the knee until your leg is nearly touching the floor.

6. Bring both arm and leg back to the starting position. Keep breathing and avoid twisting your lower back.

7. Reverse the movement, bringing your left arm and right leg down until they almost touch the floor.

8. Repeat the cycle 10 times.

STAY SAFE:

If you notice you're slipping out of the correct form, your muscles are getting tired and it's probably a good idea to finish up. There are two reasons to stop. First, without proper form, you will no longer be getting the full benefit of the exercise. Second, when using improper form, you are more likely to injure yourself. And, as always, if doing the exercise is causing pain, stop.

EASY DOES IT:

One of the big challenges of this exercise is maintaining constant contact between the floor and the lower back. If you have trouble doing so, your core needs work. One way to correct your form is to bring your arms and legs down just part of the way toward the floor. When you notice your lower back losing contact, pull back a few degrees. As you repeat the exercise, you will be able to bring your arms and legs closer to the floor while keeping your lower back pressed snugly to the floor.

Once you've mastered the easy exercises, it's time to move up to the medium program. I've structured the medium program to feel similar to the easy program so your transition is easier while you step up the difficulty. Many of these exercises are modified versions of those in the easy program, but with new wrinkles to make them more challenging and effective.

A lot of the exercises will also bring the exercise ball (or physioball) into play. You can pick up a ball relatively cheap online or at an exercise or sporting goods store. Get a ball that's the right size for you: When you lie on your back on the ball, your feet should fully rest on the floor. I recommend a ball with a 55 cm (approximately 22 inches) diameter for people under 5'8" and a ball with a 65 cm (approximately 26 inches) diameter for those who are taller.

Before you start the workout program, I recommend sitting upright on your exercise ball and bouncing gently. This movement will force you into an upright posture, engage your core, and start to get your blood pumping. It also feels good. Do it for 20 to 30 seconds before beginning any of the exercises.

BASIC PLANK

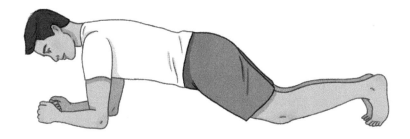

Throughout my years of practice, I have studied many traditional Eastern healing systems. And while the theories behind the various practices may seem alien to Western understanding, there are many similarities in therapeutic work.

About a decade ago, I was in the Metropolitan Museum of Art in New York City, walking around an exhibit titled "Venice and the Islamic World: 828–1797." One glass case contained a very large book, Ibn Sina's *Canon of Medicine*, the most authoritative medical text in the Islamic world at the time. On the open page was a picture of a man lying facedown on a table and another man standing above him with his hands on his back. The descriptive caption on the case read, "Doctor performing a spinal manipulation on a patient." This spinal manipulation was documented and illustrated in Persia in approximately 1000 CE.

Historical practitioners' reasoning for why joint manipulation was effective bears little resemblance to the modern physiological explanation for the effectiveness of the treatment, but the end result was surely the same.

The same is true for the plank. Yoga is part of the Indian healing tradition known as Ayurveda. Just as science has caught up with chiropractic, science is also catching up with yoga to explain why the movements are essential for building a strong and stable core and why this particular exercise is so important in preventing lower back pain.

Instructions:

1. Lie facedown on your stomach on the floor.

2. Lift yourself up so you are resting on both your knees and your forearms. Form is key!

3. Your shoulders should be directly over your elbows.

4. Focus on elongating the spine as you hold this position.

5. Try to hold for 60 seconds. It may take some time for you to get there. (See the Easy Does It note on this page for advice on ramping up to 60 seconds.)

Once you're comfortable holding for 60 seconds, modify the plank so your knees are off the floor and you're holding yourself up with your toes and forearms.

STAY SAFE:

Do not do this exercise (or any of the planks described in this book) if you are suffering from any upper extremity problems, like a shoulder, elbow, or wrist injury, particularly carpal tunnel, as you will be putting a tremendous amount of pressure on the wrist. Avoid the plank if you have any lower extremity injuries, too. This exercise puts a great deal of force through all these joints.

EASY DOES IT:

The plank is a challenging exercise, so approach it accordingly. It can take some time to get to a 60-second hold. Start out by holding for 5 to 10 seconds for the first week. Work your way up to 15- to 20-second holds during the second week, adding 10 to 15 seconds each week until you hit the magic 60-second goal. Who knows? You might want to keep going and get into planking competitions. The world record as of this writing is held by a 62-year-old former marine who held his position for 8 hours, 15 minutes, and 15 seconds!

MEDIUM

SIDE PLANK

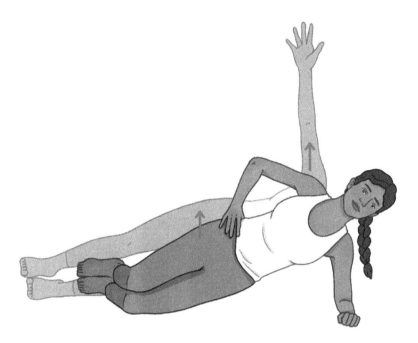

Side planks put a stronger focus on your quadratus lumborum, which is at the back of the abdominal wall and plays a huge role in preventing back pain.

Side planks are more challenging than traditional planks—it's okay if you aren't perfect on day one, but don't quit. Work your way up slowly. The benefits are worth it.

Instructions:

1. Lie faceup on the floor.

2. Turn on your side and rest on your elbow, keeping your knees bent backward at a right angle.

3. Lift your hips off the floor, maintaining a straight line from shoulders to hips to knees.

4. Try to hold for 60 seconds. It may take some time for you to get there.

Once you can hold for 60 seconds comfortably, instead of bending your knees, keep your legs straight as you lift both your knees and hips off the floor.

To increase the challenge, extend your non-supporting arm straight into the air and hold the position.

STAY SAFE:

Balance can be an issue with the side plank, especially when you lift your knees off the floor. If need be, cross one leg over the other for stability.

EASY DOES IT:

Much like the basic plank, you can work your way up to 60 seconds on the side plank. Start with 5 to 10 seconds for the first week, go for 15 to 20 seconds the second week, and add more time gradually until you're comfortably side planking for 60 seconds.

MEDIUM

MEDIUM

CRUNCH WITH EXERCISE BALL

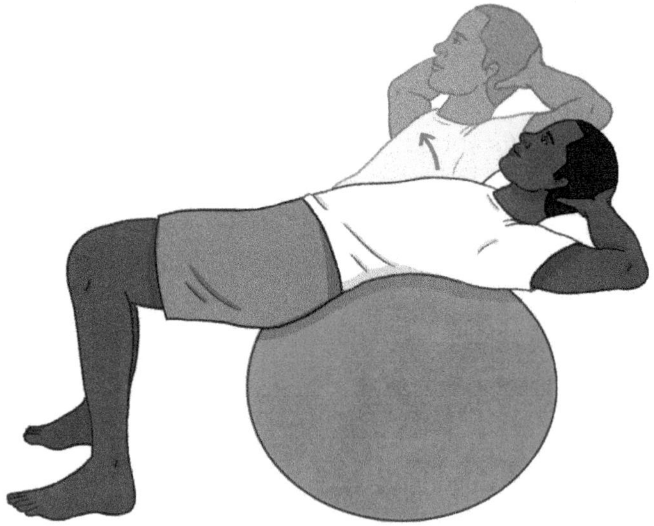

The Crunches exercise in the easy workout program (page 86) is a good way to work your abdominal muscles, but adding an exercise ball works them even more. Don't bring in the exercise ball until you've mastered crunches on the floor. You need a lot more balance on the ball, and it's quite easy to slip out of proper form (or slip and fall).

Instructions:

1. Sit upright on the exercise ball.

2. Grasp your hands together behind your neck to provide support.

3. Slowly walk forward with small steps. At the same time, lower your torso until the ball is directly beneath the arch of your lumbar spine. You want your torso and lower back in a straight line, parallel to the floor. This is called neutral position.

4. Gently drop your torso so it is lower than your hips. This is called being in negative space, meaning you're below neutral.

5. Gently lift your torso, with hands firmly behind your neck, past neutral position and up 25 to 30 degrees, into what is called positive space.

6. Come back into the negative space position and repeat the cycle 5 to 10 times.

STAY SAFE:

Always use the exercise ball on a padded surface, such as a rubber mat or a carpet. There's always a chance you might slip off the ball, so be sure you can fall onto some cushioning.

EASY DOES IT:

The amount you inflate the exercise ball affects the difficulty of the crunches. Exercises require less effort when the ball is softer than when it's rigid. When the ball is less inflated, you will sink into it more, so you will be much more stable. As you get into position, the ball will almost engulf you, making it less likely that you'll fall off. When you're starting out with the ball, you may want it in a softer state.

MEDIUM

SUPINE TWIST WITH EXERCISE BALL

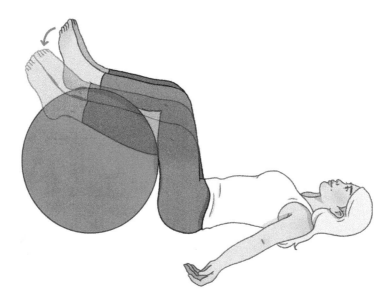

Much like the Supine Twist exercise in the easy workout (page 88), the goal with this exercise is to work the ab muscles you aren't working with the crunches: the transverse and oblique abdominals. The exercise ball increases the degree of difficulty, making the supine twist more effective, especially if your body has become accustomed to the easier variation.

Instructions:

1. Lie faceup on the floor with your legs over the exercise ball. The goal is to keep your hips and knees at approximately 90 degrees to the ball.

2. Slowly rotate your legs to the left while keeping your back in contact with the floor. You're basically rolling the ball to the left with your heels. Rotate as far as you can.

3. Slowly rotate back to the right, again keeping your back in contact with the floor. Go as far as you can.

4. Return your legs to the starting position.

5. Repeat 10 to 15 times.

STAY SAFE:

Keep your back on the floor! Not only is it important for the effectiveness of the exercise, but it also keeps you safe. Proper form is more important than rotating your legs a few degrees further.

EASY DOES IT:

You may find you can't rotate particularly far in either direction at first. That's okay. Go as far as you can. Over time, you'll become more flexible.

FACEDOWN (PRONE) BACK EXTENSION WITH EXERCISE BALL

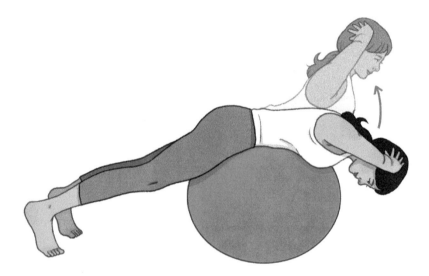

This exercise is almost like a reverse sit-up on top of an exercise ball. When done correctly, it's very effective for developing your lower back and core strength. The correct form is more challenging than anything in the easy workout program, however, so you may need some practice to get the mechanics right.

Instructions:

1. Place the exercise ball in front of you and kneel on the floor.

2. Lean on the ball with your elbows and forearms.

3. Roll forward until the ball is underneath your stomach. Balance yourself by putting your hands on the floor in front of you and keeping your feet on the floor behind you.

4. Lift your arms off the floor and bend them at the elbows so your hands are next to your head.

5. Do a reverse sit-up: Slowly raise your torso until it is parallel to the floor, and if you can, raise it another 10 to 15 degrees. You will feel the tension of your lower back muscles being activated. You may feel a bit unstable or wobbly, so if you need to, drop your arms to the floor again rather than falling off the ball.

6. Hold at the end point, then lower your torso back to the starting position.

7. Repeat 5 to 10 times.

As you become comfortable and stable with this exercise, you can raise your arms and your legs at the same time in what is known as superhero pose.

STAY SAFE:

You will know you are doing the exercise correctly if you feel the muscles in your lower back tightening because they are doing all the work. If you feel sharp pain, stop. If you can feel your gluteal (buttock), hamstring, or upper back muscles tightening, reposition yourself on the ball so movement focuses on the muscles of the lumbar spine.

EASY DOES IT:

Don't rush the exercise. It is combining strength with balance, so it may take you a bit longer to master compared to exercises that are purely for strength. Be patient. You'll get there.

MEDIUM

FACEUP (SUPINE) BACK EXTENSION WITH EXERCISE BALL

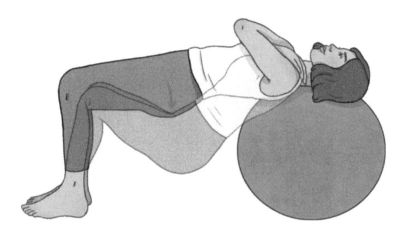

You may have used an exercise ball on your own for stretching or exercising, but I highly doubt you've ever done this exercise. It requires putting your body in an odd position, and few people will think to try without supervision. It's another good exercise for your lower back, as well as your glutes, hamstrings, quadriceps, and overall balance.

Instructions:

1. Place the exercise ball behind you and kneel on the floor, facing away from the ball.

2. Roll your back onto the exercise ball, positioning the ball underneath your upper back. You should be looking up at the ceiling.

3. Continue to slowly position your body until your knees are bent at 90 degrees and your torso and upper legs are forming a straight line. Keep your upper back on the ball.

4. Slowly lower your pelvis toward the floor, then lift back up to the 180-degree position.

5. Repeat 10 to 15 times.

STAY SAFE:

It can be *very* easy to lose your balance during this exercise, especially as you drop your pelvis, and your upper back may start to slip off the ball. Drop your pelvis only as low as you can while keeping your upper back (and the ball) in a stationary position. You won't be able to touch your buttocks to the floor on day one—or possibly ever. Go only as far as you can safely. Balance and safety are more important than a deeper stretch.

EASY DOES IT:

Go only as low as you can while keeping your upper back firmly on the ball. You may want to use a slightly softer exercise ball (see Easy Does It tip on page 107), which will improve stability.

Also, because of the rather unorthodox position of this exercise, it can be helpful to set up in front of a mirror at first so you can better gauge whether you're properly positioned.

ALTERNATING LEG BALANCE WITH BALANCE PAD

MEDIUM

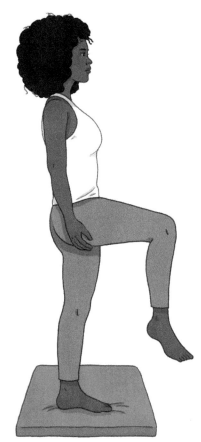

Once you have mastered the Alternating Leg Balance exercise on page 94, you can make it more challenging by adding some additional equipment. My preferred tool is the balance pad, a piece of foam padding that is about two inches thick. The foam is not uniform in density, so when you stand on it, you have to engage different muscles than when you stand on solid ground.

Instructions:

1. Place the balance pad on the floor.

2. Stand on the pad and lift one leg, bent at the knee. Your thigh should be perpendicular to the floor with your calf making a 90-degree angle.

3. Hold this position for up to 30 seconds.

4. Repeat with the other leg.

5. Once you are able to hold the position for 30 seconds on each leg, repeat the exercise with your eyes closed, until you are able to maintain balance for 30 seconds.

Once you are able to stand on the pad with your eyes closed for 30 seconds on each leg, turn the pad 90 degrees and perform the exercise again. Because of the unequal distribution of foam density, the pad will feel completely different in this new position. When you've mastered the second position and can balance on each leg for 30 seconds with your eyes closed, rotate another 90 degrees and then another, until you have covered the full pad.

With every change in rotation you will be activating different muscles, providing a greater degree of rehabilitation to all the joints of the feet and ankles.

STAY SAFE:

I discussed the risk of falling when you were doing the Alternating Leg Balance exercise in the easy workout program—and you were standing on one leg on flat ground. Now you're standing on intentionally uneven ground. Make sure you have something stable nearby to grab if you lose your balance.

EASY DOES IT:

Your first time on a balance pad will be unlike anything you've experienced. If you can't lift your leg to 90 degrees, just lift it a little. If you can't hold the position for 30 seconds, hold it as long as you can. Eventually you'll adjust to the feeling of balancing on uneven ground.

CROSS CRAWL WITH EXERCISE BALL

MEDIUM

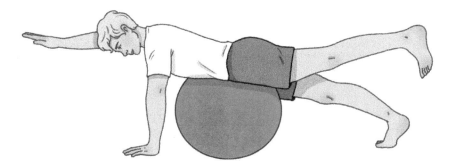

The Cross Crawl exercise on the floor (page 96) was one of the most challenging exercises in the easy workout. This variation is even more challenging, but the payoff is worth it. When you master this version of the cross crawl, you should feel your core tightening and find you are walking more upright. You may even notice you have increased energy.

Because you are forced into cat position, at first you'll do the exercise with a rounded back.

One quick note: Your exercise ball must be small enough to allow your knees and hands to touch the floor when you're on top of the ball in cat position.

Instructions:

1. Lie facedown on the ball, positioning it under your stomach. Place your hands on the floor in front of you and your knees on the floor behind you.

2. Lift your right arm in front of you.

3. Hold your arm straight out for three to five seconds.

4. Bring your hand back to the floor.

5. Do the same movement with the left arm, again holding for three to five seconds.

6. Bring your right leg straight out behind you.

7. Hold for three to five seconds.

8. Bring your knee back to the floor.

9. Do the same movement with the left leg, again holding for three to five seconds.

10. Lift the left arm and the right leg at the same time and hold for three to five seconds before returning them to the floor.

11. Lift the right arm and the left leg at the same time and hold for three to five seconds before returning them to the floor.

12. Repeat the entire sequence three times.

If your ball is soft enough, you may be able to perform the exercise in cow position. But if it's not, you will still get a great deal of benefit.

You can also modify this exercise using two foam rollers. Place one roller underneath your knees and the other underneath your hands, and perform the exercise as described above.

STAY SAFE:

When you have one arm out and one leg up, you're really relying on your other arm, other leg, and core strength to keep you balanced on the ball. If you start to tip over, bring your leg back down for stability. Your instinct may be to put your hand down first, but doing so could cause you to jam or even sprain your wrist if you hit the floor incorrectly.

EASY DOES IT:

Work your way up to the final steps of the one arm up, one leg up positions. As with many of the exercises that use the ball, a softer ball will provide more stability.

DEAD BUG WITH FOAM ROLLER

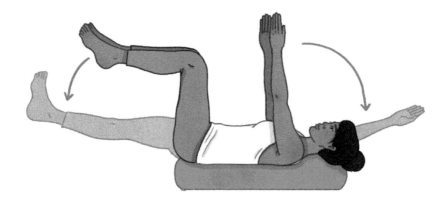

We're going to increase the challenge of the Dead Bug (page 98) by bringing a foam roller into the mix. This exercise will be your biggest balance challenge in the medium workout program. You have to keep your core muscles engaged for the entire exercise or you'll roll right off the foam roller.

Instructions:

1. Put a long foam roller on the floor and lie on top of it, faceup, so the foam roller is supporting the length of your spine.

2. Keep your arms on the floor as you bring both knees up, bending them at 90-degree angles.

3. Bring both arms up straight. If you find it impossible to balance in this position, keep your left arm on the floor for a bit of stability.

4. Slowly bring your right arm down so it's nearly touching the ground. Your arm should be aligned with your body with your palm facing up.

5. At the same time, bring your left leg down, extending the knee until your leg is nearly touching the floor.

6. Bring both arm and leg back to the starting position. It is important to keep breathing and avoid twisting your lower back.

7. Reverse the movement, bringing your left arm and right leg down until they almost touch the floor.

8. Repeat the cycle 10 times.

STAY SAFE:

Balance is a real challenge with this exercise. Keep one arm on the floor to improve your stability if you need to; otherwise, you may find yourself rolling onto the floor once you start moving your arms and legs.

EASY DOES IT:

While the ideal form of this exercise involves simultaneous arm and leg movements, you can do the arm exercises alone and then the leg exercises alone until you're ready to take them on concurrently.

MEDIUM

Congratulations! The medium program is *not* easy. But you mastered it, and now you're ready to take on some really challenging core exercises. While some of them involve just your body weight, others will employ the exercise ball, a foam roller, or a pull-up bar.

Warning: These exercises are not for the faint of heart—or body. But if you can complete the workout successfully, you'll have a strong, well-trained core that should do wonders protecting you from back pain.

CLIMBING PLANK

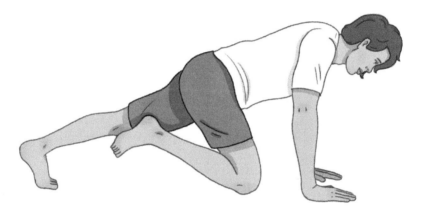

You're going to do three—yes, *three*—versions of the plank (page 102) in this workout. The plank is one of the foundational core exercises (the core-core exercises, if you will), and the better you get at doing all the variations, the more your back will thank you.

The first plank in the advanced workout is the climbing plank, also referred to as the mountain climber. You'll begin in a position similar to a traditional plank, but you won't stay there long.

Instructions:

1. Get on the floor in a plank position, supporting the top part of your body with your hands or forearms. (See the "Easy Does It" note).

2. Bring your right knee forward toward your chest while keeping your other leg straight. This is called the climbing plank because you're performing the motion you'd use to hike up a mountain or a set of stairs.

3. Return to the starting position.

4. Perform the same exercise with the left knee.

5. Repeat 5 to 10 times.

STAY SAFE:

Avoid bouncing your hips up and down as you perform the climbing motion so you maintain effectiveness and safety. You may see videos on YouTube of people doing intense, incredibly fast mountain climbers where it looks like they're trying to sprint up an imaginary horizontal version of Mount Everest. You don't need to do that. Go slow and choose form over speed.

EASY DOES IT:

You can position yourself with your hands or your forearms on the floor. If you're on your forearms, the exercise will be a bit easier, as your forearms will give you more stability and put less strain on your shoulders. But if you're on your hands, you'll be able to get a better range of motion. If you have long legs, you'll probably need to be on your hands to keep your knees from hitting the floor.

PLANK WITH LEG EXTENSIONS

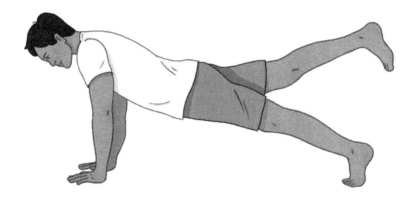

The plank with leg extensions works your lower back, plus your abdominals, quadriceps, glutes, shoulders, chest, and triceps. While some of these muscle groups are outside the scope of your lower back pain workout regimen, I'm sure you won't mind toning them in the process.

Instructions:

1. Get on the floor in a plank position, supporting the top part of your body with your hands or forearms. Much like the climber plank, forearms are a little easier, but hands give you a more thorough workout (and engage your shoulder and arm muscles even more).

2. Lift your right foot off the floor, extending your leg up toward the ceiling.

3. Drop your leg to return to starting position.

4. Lift your left foot off the floor, extending your leg up toward the ceiling.

5. Drop your leg to return to starting position.

6. Repeat 5 to 10 times.

STAY SAFE:

Throughout the exercise, squeeze your abdominal muscles to protect your back, and make sure to keep your body as close to parallel to the floor as possible.

EASY DOES IT:

Your range of motion may be limited, especially at first. Keep your leg straight as you lift it up—resist the temptation to bend your knees. You'll work your way up to greater height.

STAGGERED PLANK

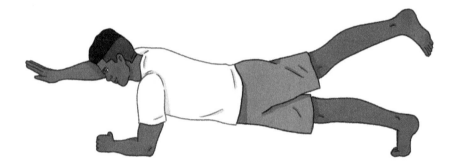

Warning: This is the most difficult of the five planks in this book. Don't jump right into it. You'll need the strong core and improved balance you've developed from the easy and medium workouts to carry you through.

Instructions:

1. Get on the floor in a plank position, supporting the top part of your body with your forearms. You may also use your hands, but using your forearms is easier.

2. Extend your left arm out in front of you as you simultaneously lift your right leg and extend it out behind you.

3. Hold for five seconds, then return to starting position.

4. Perform the same motion with your right arm and left leg.

5. Repeat the cycle 5 to 10 times.

STAY SAFE:

It's easy to lose your balance during this exercise, especially if you aren't engaging your core. Keep your abdominal muscles tight, and if you start wobbling during one of the five-second holds, cut it short and bring your arm and leg down to stabilize your body.

EASY DOES IT:

If you find it too challenging to extend both your arm and leg at the same time, extend your arm first, then your leg. And, as with the other planks, you can find more stability by positioning yourself on your forearms rather than your hands.

CROSS CLIMBER

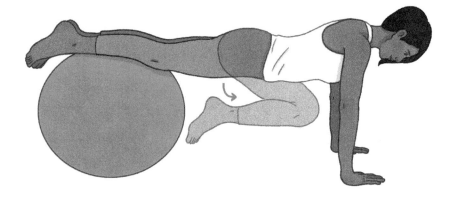

I know what you're thinking: Phew, not another plank. Well . . . although it may not *technically* be a plank, the cross climber has a lot of plank-like characteristics. Call it a first cousin of the plank. This exercise is a thorough core and back workout, and as an added bonus, it will help you strengthen your chest and shoulders.

Set aside 60 to 90 seconds between completing the last exercise and beginning this one. Drink some water, remember to breathe, then jump back in.

Instructions:

1. Place the exercise ball in front of you and lie on top of it, facedown.

2. Put your hands flat on the floor and walk them forward until you're in a push-up position with your shins on the exercise ball. Form a straight line with your body from your back to your feet.

3. Lift your right leg off the ball and, with your knee bent, bring your knee toward your left elbow. Keep your lower back straight, not rounded, throughout the motion.

4. Bring your knee back to your starting position with both shins on the ball.

5. Repeat the motion with the other side, bringing your left knee toward your right elbow.

6. Do five repetitions on each side.

STAY SAFE:

This exercise also requires a padded floor, as you have a good chance of falling from the ball to the floor at some point.

EASY DOES IT:

Go slow. You have a lot to think about: keeping your body straight, avoiding rounding your back, moving one knee toward the opposite elbow. You're not in a race. Take your time and focus on form over speed.

HARD

JACKKNIFE WITH PUSH-UP

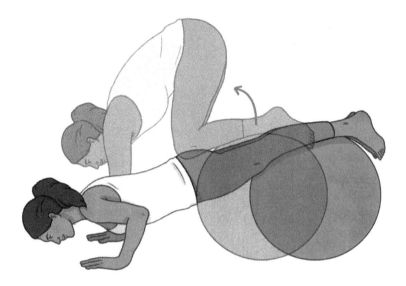

This is another exercise where you'll be in the push-up position with your legs on the exercise ball. But this time you're actually going to do the push-ups. This exercise challenges your strength, balance, and coordination.

Instructions:

1. Start in the same position as you did in the Cross Climber exercise (page 128): push-up position, shins on the exercise ball, back flat.

2. Do a push-up, lowering your torso as close to the floor as possible, then come back up to the starting position.

3. Pull the exercise ball toward your chest with your feet and shins by bending your knees. Make sure to keep your back straight and tighten your abs.

4. Hold the position for three to five seconds, then roll the ball back with your feet and shins to the starting point.

5. Repeat the process (push-up, followed by pulling in the ball) five times.

STAY SAFE:

Balance is of paramount importance in this exercise. If you start wobbling, lower yourself slowly to the floor. It's a much better option than falling face-first or to the side.

EASY DOES IT:

When I instruct you to "pull the exercise ball toward your chest," the emphasis is on *toward*. You will use your legs and core strength to bring the ball forward, but it's not going to make it all the way to your chest, even once you're an expert. That might not even be humanly possible. Roll the ball forward as far as you can and work your way up to greater distance.

EXERCISE BALL PUSH-UP

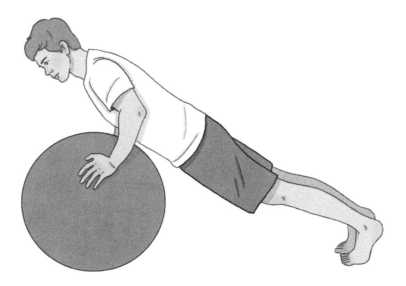

You've now done two consecutive exercises in a push-up position with your feet on the exercise ball. For this exercise, you're going to do more push-ups, but with your arms on the exercise ball rather than your legs. You'll rely heavily on your core to keep yourself stable during the push-ups, because they are *not* easy.

Instructions:

1. Place the exercise ball in front of you.

2. Put your hands on the ball and get into a push-up position. Your shoulders should be above the center of the ball and your elbows should be straight. Your back should be a straight line.

3. Slowly bend your elbows and lower your chest toward the ball.

4. When your chest touches the ball, slowly push back up.

5. Repeat 5 to 10 times.

STAY SAFE:

Make sure you feel totally balanced on the ball before you begin doing the push-ups. You don't want to start dropping your chest down when you're unbalanced, have the ball pop out from underneath you, and crash face-first onto the floor.

EASY DOES IT:

A deflated ball definitely reduces the difficulty in this exercise. The more your hands can sink into the ball, the less you'll have to stabilize yourself throughout the movement.

HARD

ALTERNATING LEG BALANCE WITH ROCKER BOARD OR FOAM ROLLER

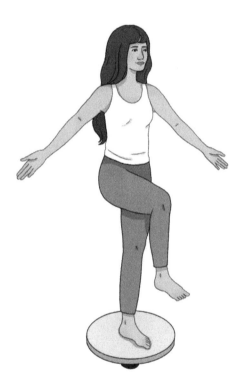

You'll scale up the difficulty of leg balancing once again. But at least no planks or push-ups are involved!

For this variation on the Alternating Leg Balance exercise (page 94), you'll incorporate either a rocker board or a foam roller.

A rocker board is a carpet-covered square plank atop two rounded (half-moon) legs. When you stand on the board or foam roller, you will feel wobbly. But when you successfully complete the exercises, you will have achieved true stability of your feet and ankles, thus eliminating a downstream cause of your lower back pain.

Instructions:

For the rocker board:

1. Place the rocker board on the floor.

2. Stand on top of it and get yourself balanced.

3. Stand on one leg and hold the position for 30 seconds. Once you can do it with your eyes open, do it with your eyes closed.

4. Rotate 90 degrees and repeat the process.

For the foam roller:

1. Place the roller on the floor and stand on top of it, with the roller horizontally positioned under your feet. Your feet should be shoulder-width apart. It's best to do this in bare feet or socks so your feet can wrap around the roller.

2. Get balanced. It's tough!

3. Bend your knees into a half squat.

4. Raise your arms in front of you, forming a 90-degree angle with your body.

5. Hold the position for three to five seconds.

6. To make the exercise more challenging, do it while raising one leg, then the other.

STAY SAFE:

You will very likely fall off the board or roller while doing these master-level balancing exercises. Do the exercises next to something stable you can grab if you feel yourself starting to go down.

EASY DOES IT:

It can be hard to find your balance on top of the rocker board or foam roller, even after you've been working at the exercises for some time. You can make the process easier by holding onto a chair or other sturdy item as you step on the unstable item and find your balance. Slowly let go only once you feel you're balanced.

HANGING LEG RAISE

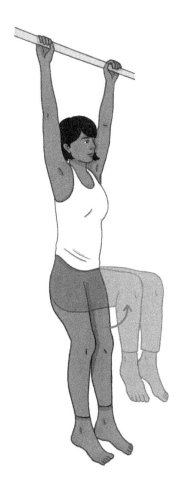

It is now time to incorporate the pull-up bar into your workout routine.
    The hanging leg raise makes me think of the gymnastics competitions at the Olympics. I marvel at the incredible core strength of these world-class athletes as they swing on the high bars or rings. And although you may just be hanging from a pull-up bar at the neighborhood playground, you can feel the same burn in your abs.

Instructions:

1. Hang from the pull-up bar with your palms facing forward.

2. Slowly bring your knees up toward your chest. Do not lean your torso backward.

3. When you have brought your knees as high as you can, do a crunch, tucking your knees into your chest.

4. Slowly lower your legs, being mindful to control the movement and engage your abs.

5. Repeat the cycle 10 times.

You'll know you have elite core strength when you can add on a move to this exercise called the front lever. That's where you lift up your entire body while hanging from the bar, so you're completely parallel to the ground.

STAY SAFE:

Make sure you have a really good grip on the bar before you begin. You may want to invest in weight-lifting gloves to improve your grip. They aren't expensive, and they can help you maintain a safer hold.

If you're setting up your pull-up bar in a doorway in your home, make sure it's *firmly* in the doorjamb. If the bar comes down while you're hanging, you could be seriously injured.

EASY DOES IT:

If you're doing the exercise at a gym, you may see an alternative apparatus you can use to make it easier to start. Rather than hanging from a bar, you place your forearms on a padded surface and let your body hang. This variation requires far less strength and balance, but it can help you learn the motion as you work your way up to the pull-up bar.

HARD

BANANA ROLL

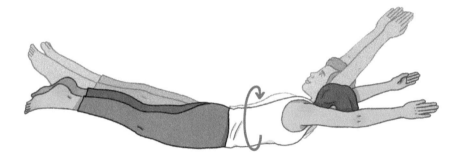

For the last exercise of this book, you will go back to the floor and ditch all the extra tools, using only your body weight and core muscles.

Many of my patients love the gym, but I also have plenty who can't stand it. They don't enjoy being around lots of sweaty people, and they feel bored and maybe self-conscious. But they still want to exercise. I tell my gym-hating patients that they don't have to join a gym—they already belong to one.

When look puzzled, I tell them to gaze outside, where they can just head out the door and start walking. Then I ask them if they have a floor. "What?" they respond. I tell them that if they have a floor in their home or in their office, then they have a place where they can stretch their bodies using only their body weight and, if they like, a few very inexpensive tools, like an exercise ball and a foam roller.

Instructions:

1. Lie on your stomach in superhero position: arms straight out in front and legs straight out behind you, all of them lifted toward the ceiling, arching your lower back.

2. Using only your abdominal muscles, not engaging your hip muscles, wriggle from side to side until you are able to flip over so you are lying on your back.

3. Flatten your lower back against the floor.

4. Hold the position for three to five seconds.

5. If you've dropped your arms and legs, bring them off the floor while you press and balance on your flexed lower back.

6. Using your core muscles (again, not your hip muscles), roll side to side, until you are able to tip yourself back over onto your stomach.

7. Hold the position for three to five seconds.

8. Repeat the cycle five times.

STAY SAFE:

The rolling-over motion should be smooth and natural. Don't kick with your leg to flip your body. Not only does that motion negate many of the benefits to your core, but jerking also puts you at a higher risk of feeling a tweak in your body.

EASY DOES IT:

It can be tricky to keep your arms and legs elevated throughout the entire rolling motion. You may feel them dropping. That's not the ideal form of the exercise, but it can help you as you adjust and grow your expertise.

HARD

Epilogue

There is a good chance that if you read this book, you have had back pain at some point in your lifetime. I hope you've learned that you can do so much to help yourself through an episode of pain. More important, you've learned there is so much you can do to prevent the pain from returning.

Many treatments are available today, from chiropractic to acupuncture to physical therapy, to help relieve back pain. Each has its strengths and weaknesses. However, what is universally agreed upon across all disciplines is that exercise should be a part of any therapeutic approach. Often, it is the only treatment you need.

When patients come to see me with pain, they are seeking relief. And I tell them that is the *first* order of business. However, I let them know it's ultimately more important to figure out the root causes *behind* their pain and to give them the tools so they can help heal themselves at that time and, if necessary, again in the future.

If you are working at a nonergonomic workstation which is causing you to sit with bad posture day after day and year after year and contributing to your pain and dysfunction, I recommend ergonomic and behavioral changes. If your job involves repetitive lifting of heavy objects, learn the proper lifting form (and again, don't let your back muscles go soft by relying on lumbar support).

Regardless of your line of work, the single most important measure to prevent back pain is a strong and stable core, as all your movement, power, and balance emanates from your core.

That's what this book is all about. Of course, there are situations when you may need the help of a health-care professional, especially if you have symptoms like radiating leg pain or numbness or pain that is just too debilitating to handle on your own. But even then, you may find the most effective treatment is exercise.

Finally, now that you have the tools at your fingertips, you need to use them. The more you do, the less I, or any other health-care practitioner, have to do. It's your call.

Go forth and exercise! Do your cardio, stretch those muscles, and work that core. The power to heal is in your hands. And in your back!

Resources

I have found that understanding the causes of my patients' complaints, educating them about those causes, and giving them the tools to support their own healing has been one of the most satisfying parts of my work. Holistic care is about looking at the many possible contributors to a person's state of health: mechanical, chemical, and emotional. If you would like to explore more deeply, I suggest you consider the following resources:

DeFlame.com
The website of Dr. David Seaman, MS, DC. He is the author of *The DeFlame Diet*, the first in a series of excellent books that describe the relationship between food, pain, and chronic disease.

McKenzieInstituteUSA.org
A website dedicated to the work of Robin McKenzie, a New Zealand physical therapist, who developed a series of protocols used to determine exercises that can be very effective for treating back pain, especially pain related to disc dysfunctions.

BackFitPro.com
A website featuring the work of Stuart McGill, PhD, one of the world's leading researchers on the relationship between back pain and exercise.

ConditionHealthNews.com
Dr. Ricky Fishman's health news and information website features cutting-edge stories by Dr. Fishman and other experts on back care, health and wellness, ergonomics, and more.

TheBackSchool.net
This resource is great for ergonomics information, including product reviews, classes, and great healthy back tips.

NIA.NIH.gov

The National Institute on Aging, which is part of the U.S. National Institutes of Health, is a great source of healthy tips for those aged 50 and older. Their website includes exercises, videos, health information, and tracking tools to support workouts.

MindfulnessCDs.com

Jon Kabat-Zinn is a professor of medicine and the creator of the mindfulness-based stress reduction (MBSR) program. His first book, of many, was *Full Catastrophe Living*. He teaches meditation techniques that can help people cope with stress, anxiety, pain, and illness.

References

American Chiropractic Association, n.d. "Back Pain Facts and Statistics." ACAToday.
org/Patients/What-is-Chiropractic/Back-Pain-Facts-and-Statistics.

Cleveland Clinic. n.d. "Chronic Back Pain." my.ClevelandClinic.org/health
/diseases/16869-chronic-back-pain.

———. n.d. "Spine Structure & Function." my.ClevelandClinic.org/health/articles
/10040-spine-structure-and-function.

DeFlame. 2020. "DeFlame Enterprise: DeFlaming Supplements." DeFlame.com.

Johns Hopkins Medicine, n.d. "Intermittent Fasting: What Is It, and How Does It
Work?" HopkinsMedicine.org/health/wellness-and-prevention/intermittent
-fasting-what-is-it-and-how-does-it-work.

Mayo Foundation for Medical Education and Research. 2020. "Back Pain."
MayoClinic.org/diseases-conditions/back-pain/diagnosis-treatment
/drc-20369911.

The Metropolitan Museum of Art, n.d. "Venice and the Islamic World, 828–1797."
MetMuseum.org/exhibitions/listings/2007/venice-and-the-islamic-world.

Office of Environment, Health and Safety, University of California San Francisco.
n.d. "Maintain a Neutral Posture." EHS.UCSF.edu/maintain-neutral-posture.

Robertson, David, Dinesh Kumbhare, Paul Nolet, John Srbely, and Genevieve Newton. 2017. "Associations between Low Back Pain and Depression and Somatization in a Canadian Emerging Adult Population." *The Journal of the Canadian Chiropractic Association* 61(2): 96–105. NCBI.NLM.NIH.gov/pmc /articles/PMC5596967.

U.S. National Library of Medicine. 2019. "Low Back Pain: Why Movement Is So Important for Back Pain." NCBI.NLM.NIH.gov/books/NBK284944.

WebMD. 2020. "Back Surgery: Pros and Cons." WebMD.com/back-pain /back-surgery-types.

Index

A

Acupuncture, 23
Acute pain, 3
Adductor muscles, 66–67
Age, as a risk factor, 14
American Chiropractic Association, 2
Anatomy, 6–9
Ayurveda, 23

B

Back anatomy, 6–9
Back pain
    causes of, 2–3, 9–12
    diagnosing, 17–20
    emotions and, 12–13
    prevalence of, 2
    prevention, 25–26
    risk factors, 13–14
    treatment options, 20–25
    types of, 3
Back support belts, 26
Balance pads, 76
Blood tests, 20
Body mass index (BMI), 37
Body mechanics, 32–36
Bone scans, 20
Breathing exercises, 12–13, 26
Bulging discs, 9, 11

C

Cardio exercise, 30–32
    workouts, 45–49
Cartilage, 9
Chiropractic treatment, 22
Chronic pain, 3
Circulation, 30–31
Coccyx, 6

Computer axial tomography
    (CAT/CT scan), 20
Core strength, 43–44, 72–73.
    See also Strengthening exercises

D

Diet and nutrition, 37–38
Discography, 20
Disc replacement, 25
Discs, 6, 9, 11

E

Emergency room, when to go, 10
Emotions, and back pain, 12–13, 14
Equipment, 73, 76–77
Ergonomics, 25, 34–36
Exercise
    cardio, 30–32
    goals of, 41
    for seniors, 74–75
    strengthening–easy program, 77–100
    strengthening–hard program, 120–139
    strengthening–medium
        program, 101–119
    stretching, 51–69
    tools, 73, 76–77
    workouts, 45–49
Exercise balls, 73

F

Fight-or-flight response, 12–13
Fitness levels, 13
Foam rollers, 76
Forest bathing, 13

G

Genetics, 14
Gluteal muscles, 54 55

H

Hamstring muscles, 62–63
Herniated discs, 9, 11
High heels, and potential for
    back pain, 34

I

Infections, 10
Inflammation, 11, 12, 24, 37–38
Inflatable cushions, 77
Injuries, 32–33
Intermittent fasting, 38
Intervertebral joint complex, 7, 9, 52

J

Joints, 7, 9, 52

K

Kidney infections, 10

L

Laminectomy, 24
Laundry, and potential for back pain, 33
Leg pain, 30
Lifting, 26
Ligaments, 7, 9

M

Magnetic resonance imaging (MRI), 20
Medical imaging, 18–20
Medications, 21
Medicine balls, 77
Meditation, 13
Mental health, 14
Mind-body connection, 12–13
Motor nerves, 7
Movement. *See* Exercise
Muscles, 6–7, 9
Myelography, 20

N

Nerves, 7, 11–12
Neutral posture, 33

O

Obesity, 14, 36–38
Occupational risk, 13–14
Osteopathy, 22

P

Palmer, Daniel David, 22
Pelvis, 6
Physical exams, 17–18
Physical therapy, 22
Pinched nerves, 11–12
Piriformis muscles, 68–69
Piriformis syndrome, 11
Posture, 30, 32–36
Pregnancy, 14
Preventive tips, 25–26
Psoas muscles, 60–61
Pull-up bars, 76

Q

Quadriceps muscles, 64–65

R

Resistance bands, 76–77
Risk factors, 13–14
Rolf, Ida, 23
Rolfing, 23

S

Sacroiliac joint, 6
Sacrum, 6
Sciatica, 11
Self-massagers, 76
Seniors, exercises for, 74–75
Sensory nerves, 7
Sitting, 33–36
Sleeping habits, 34
Spinal column, 6, 30
Spinal fusion, 24
Spondylosis, 9
Sprains, 11
Stenosis, 9
Still, Andrew Taylor, 22

Strains, 11
Strengthening exercises
   alternating leg balance, 94–95
   alternating leg balance with
      balance pad, 114–115
   alternating leg balance with rocker
      board or foam roller, 134–135
   banana roll, 138–139
   basic plank, 102–103
   cat/cow, 78–79
   climbing plank, 122–123
   core strength, 43–44, 72–73
   cross climber, 128–129
   the cross crawl, 96–97
   cross crawl with exercise ball, 116–117
   the crunch, 86–87
   crunch with exercise ball, 106–107
   curl-up, 82–83
   dead bug, 98–100
   dead bug with foam roller, 118–119
   easy program, 78–100
   exercise ball push-up, 132–133
   facedown (prone) back extension,
      90–91
   facedown (prone) back extension
      with exercise ball, 110–111
   faceup (supine) back extension, 92–93
   faceup (supine) back extension
      with exercise ball, 112–113
   hanging leg raise, 136–137
   hard program, 120–139
   jackknife with push-up, 130–131
   knee-to-chest stretch, 80–81
   medium program, 101–119
   pelvic tilts, 80–81
   plank with leg extensions, 124–125
   press-up/modified cobra, 84–85
   side plank, 104–105
   staggered plank, 126–127
   supine twist, 88–89
   supine twist with exercise ball, 108–109
   tools, 73, 76–77
   workouts, 45–49, 77

Stress, 12–13
Stretching
   butterfly adductors stretch, 66–67
   hamstring doorway stretch, 62–63
   importance of, 45, 52–53
   lying leg rest piriformis stretch, 68–69
   pigeon glute stretch, 54–55
   as prevention, 25–26
   psoas doorway stretch, 60–61
   standing quadriceps stretch, 64–65
   TFL foam rolling, 58–59
   TFL wall stretch, 56–57
   workouts, 45–49
Subacute pain, 3
Supplements, 38
Surgery, 24–25

T

Tendons, 6–7
Tensor fasciae latae (TFL), 56–59
Traditional Chinese Medicine (TCM), 23
Traumatic injuries, 11
Treatment options
   acute vs. chronic pain, 20–21
   medications, 21
   noninvasive, 22–24
   surgery, 24–25
Tumors, 10

V

Vertebrae, 6, 9

W

Weight, 14, 36–38
Weights, 77
Workouts, 45–49
Workstations, 34–36

X

X-rays, 18–20

Y

Yoga, 23–24

Acknowledgments

I want to first thank Jenny Croghan, VP of Editorial Production at Callisto Media, for giving me the opportunity to write this book. After many conversations, she offered me the perfect vehicle to channel my experience. And to my two great editors, Sean Newcott and Sam Greenspan, who helped shape my words without losing my voice. And to the wonderful teachers, mentors, and colleagues I have had through the years: Gary Jacob, DC, who taught me the McKenzie Protocols; Malik Slosberg, DC, whose work as a researcher showed me the importance of integrating exercise into my practice; and John Scaringe, DC, EdD, president of the Southern California University of Health Sciences, who has supported my ideas and writing through the years. I also want to thank David Seaman, MA, DC, whose pioneering work on nutrition and inflammation helped expand my understanding of the relationships between food, lifestyle, and pain. My thanks also go out to Steven Gest, MD, Director of Emeryville Occupational Medical Center. While working as part of his integrative team and collaborating on patients, I learned so much about the effective integration of medicine, chiropractic, physical therapy, and more. And to my partner of more than 30 years at Chiromedica, Barbara Rinkoff, DC, with whom I have shared endless conversations, both personal and clinical, that have helped to shape both my philosophy and my practice. And finally, I must acknowledge my wife, Cindy Charles, who has been endlessly supportive of my writing and my work.

About the Author

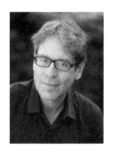

Ricky Fishman, DC, has been a doctor of chiropractic since 1986 and co-director of Chiromedica, a holistic health-care center, since 1988. There, he has brought together and assimilated the work of chiropractors, medical doctors, acupuncturists, nurse practitioners, physical therapists, and others. His philosophy of practice embraces the whole being of each person.

He is the founder of the health news and information website *Condition: Health News That Matters*, which hosts his blog and podcast and features original, cutting-edge stories by leaders in the field of integrative medicine.

In addition to working in the private health-care system, he has been staff chiropractor at Emeryville Occupational Medical Center, part of a team treating industrial injuries, since 2002. He also worked in the public health system at the Haight Ashbury Free Clinics, from 1986 to 2001, as part of a coalition of practitioners treating the uninsured of San Francisco.

To complement his clinical work, Dr. Fishman was a college professor. He taught for more than 20 years at New College of California; his courses included "Contemporary Health Studies," "Power, Politics, and Healing," "History and Philosophy of Science and Medicine," and many others. After New College he spent three years teaching "Complementary and Integrative Medicine" at the California Institute of Integral Studies in San Francisco.

Dr. Fishman is also an electric bass player who has performed with many Bay Area bands since the punk rock days of 1970s San Francisco. He has a special interest in treating musicians and other performing artists. This led him to founding the Musicians Chiropractic Project, a program that is dedicated to the specific health-care needs of working artists.